Underground Clinical Vignettes

Biochemistry

FIFTH EDITION

Underground Clinical Vignettes

Biochemistry

FIFTH EDITION

Todd A. Swanson, M.D., Ph.D.
Resident in Radiation Oncology
William Beaumont Hospital
Royal Oak, Michigan

Sandra I. Kim, M.D., Ph.D.
Resident in Internal Medicine
Beth Israel Deaconess Medical Center
Harvard Medical School
Boston, Massachusetts

Marc J. Glucksman, Ph.D.
Professor of Biochemistry and Molecular Biology
Director, Midwest Proteome Center and
Co-Director, Rosalind Franklin Structural Biology Laboratories
Rosalind Franklin University of Medicine and Science
The Chicago Medical School
North Chicago, Illinois

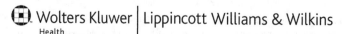

Wolters Kluwer | Lippincott Williams & Wilkins
Health

Philadelphia · Baltimore · New York · London
Buenos Aires · Hong Kong · Sydney · Tokyo

Acquisitions Editor: Nancy Anastasi Duffy
Developmental Editor: Kathleen H. Scogna
Managing Editor: Nancy Hoffmann
Marketing Manager: Jennifer Kuklinski
Associate Production Manager: Kevin P. Johnson
Creative Director: Doug Smock
Compositor: International Typesetting and Composition
Printer: R.R. Donnelley & Son's—Crawfordsville

Printed in the United States of America

First Edition, 2001 Blackwell Publishing Inc.
Second Edition, 2003 Blackwell Publishing Inc.
Third Edition, 2005 Blackwell Publishing Inc.
Fourth Edition, 2005 Blackwell Publishing Inc.

Library of Congress Cataloging-in-Publication Data

Swanson, Todd A.
   Biochemistry / Todd Swanson, Sandra Kim, Marc J. Glucksman.—5th ed.
       p. ; cm.—(Underground clinical vignettes)
   Rev. ed. of: Biochemistry / Vikas Bhushan . . . [et al.]. 4th ed. c2005.
   Includes bibliographical references and index.
   ISBN-13: 978-0-7817-6472-8
   ISBN-10: 0-7817-6472-6
   1. Clinical biochemistry—Case studies.   2. Clinical
biochemistry—Examinations, questions, etc.   I. Kim, Sandra.   II. Glucksman,
Marc J.   III. Biochemistry.   IV. Title.   V. Series.
   [DNLM: 1. Biochemistry—Case Reports.   2. Biochemistry—Problems
and Exercises.   QU 18.2 S972b 2006]
    RB112.5.B48 2006
    572.8'076—dc22

                       2006100527

07 08 09 10
1 2 3 4 5 6 7 8 9 10

dedications

preface

First published in 1999, the *Underground Clinical Vignettes* (UCV) series has provided thousands of students with a highly effective review tool as they prepare for medical exams, particularly the USMLE Step 1 and 2 exams. Designed as a quick study guide, each UCV book contains patient-centered clinical cases that highlight a range of medical diagnoses.

With this new edition of UCV, we have incorporated feedback from medical students across the country to provide updated cases with expanded treatment and discussion sections. A new format enables readers to formulate an initial diagnosis prior to reading the answer, while the added differential diagnosis section encourages critical thinking about comparable cases. The inclusion of relevant MRI images, x-rays, and photographs allows students to more readily visualize the physical presentation of each case. Breakout boxes, tables, and algorithms have been added, along with all new Board format QAs, making this edition of UCV an ideal source of information for exam review, classroom discussion, or clinical rotations.

The clinical vignettes in this series are designed to give added emphasis to pathogenesis, epidemiology, management, and complications. Although each case tends to present all the signs, symptoms, and diagnostic findings for a particular illness, patients generally will not present with such a "complete" picture either clinically or on a medical examination. Cases are not meant to simulate a potential real patient or an exam vignette.

Access to LWW's online companion site, ThePoint, will be offered as a premium with the purchase of the Underground Clinical Vignettes Step 1 bundle. Benefits include an online test link and additional new Board format questions covering all UCV subject areas.

We hope you will find the UCV series informative and useful. We welcome any feedback, suggestions, or corrections you have about this series. Please contact us at LWW.com/medstudent.

contributors

Series Editors

Todd A. Swanson, M.D., Ph.D.
Resident in Radiation Oncology
William Beaumont Hospital
Royal Oak, Michigan

Sandra I. Kim, M.D., Ph.D.
Resident in Internal Medicine
Beth Israel Deaconess Medical Center
Harvard Medical School
Boston, Massachusetts

Series Contributors

Olga E. Flomin, M.D.
Resident in Obstetrics and Gynecology
William Beaumont Hospital
Royal Oak, Michigan

Medina C. Kushen, M.D.
Resident in Neurosurgery
University of Chicago Hospitals
Chicago, Illinois

Marc J. Glucksman, Ph.D.
Professor of Biochemistry and Molecular Biology
Director, Midwest Proteome Center and
Co-Director, Rosalind Franklin Structural Biology Laboratories
Rosalind Franklin University of Medicine and Science
The Chicago Medical School
North Chicago, Illinois

acknowledgments

Thanks to Dr. Alvaro Martinez, Dr. Larry Kestin and the entire radiation oncology program at William Beaumont Hospital for allowing the flexibility to work on this project during an already vigorous residency training program.

—Todd A. Swanson

Thanks to Todd for his work on this series.

—Sandra I. Kim

M.J.G. would like to thank his colleagues for suggestions during this endeavor in medical education. This tome could not be accomplished without the thousands of students taught in classes and mentored over the last 20 years at three of the finest medical schools. I would also like to especially thank two of my recent and most brilliant students . . . my coauthors.

—Marc J. Glucksman

abbreviations

ABGs	arterial blood gases	BPH	benign prostatic hypertrophy
ABPA	allergic bronchopulmonary aspergillosis	BUN	blood urea nitrogen
		CABG	coronary artery bypass grafting
ACA	anticardiolipin antibody	CAD	coronary artery disease
ACE	angiotensin-converting enzyme	CaEDTA	calcium edetate
ACL	anterior cruciate ligament	CALLA	common acute lymphoblastic leukemia antigen
ACTH	adrenocorticotropic hormone		
AD	adjustment disorder	cAMP	cyclic adenosine monophosphate
ADA	adenosine deaminase		
ADD	attention deficit disorder	C-ANCA	cytoplasmic antineutrophil cytoplasmic antibody
ADH	antidiuretic hormone		
ADHD	attention deficit hyperactivity disorder	CBC	complete blood count
		CBD	common bile duct
ADP	adenosine diphosphate	CCU	cardiac care unit
AFO	ankle-foot orthosis	CD	cluster of differentiation
AFP	α-fetoprotein	2-CdA	2-chlorodeoxyadenosine
AIDS	acquired immunodeficiency syndrome	CEA	carcinoembryonic antigen
		CFTR	cystic fibrosis transmembrane conductance regulator
ALL	acute lymphocytic leukemia		
ALS	amyotrophic lateral sclerosis	cGMP	cyclic guanosine monophosphate
ALT	alanine aminotransferase		
AML	acute myelogenous leukemia	CHF	congestive heart failure
ANA	antinuclear antibody	CK	creatine kinase
Angio	angiography	CK-MB	creatine kinase, MB fraction
AP	anteroposterior	CLL	chronic lymphocytic leukemia
APKD	adult polycystic kidney disease	CML	chronic myelogenous leukemia
aPTT	activated partial thromboplastin time	CMV	cytomegalovirus
		CN	cranial nerve
ARDS	adult respiratory distress syndrome	CNS	central nervous system
		COPD	chronic obstructive pulmonary disease
5-ASA	5-aminosalicylic acid		
ASCA	antibodies to *Saccharomyces cerevisiae*	COX	cyclooxygenase
		CP	cerebellopontine
ASO	antistreptolysin O	CPAP	continuous positive airway pressure
AST	aspartate aminotransferase		
ATLL	adult T-cell leukemia/lymphoma	CPK	creatine phosphokinase
ATPase	adenosine triphosphatase	CPPD	calcium pyrophosphate dihydrate
AV	arteriovenous, atrioventricular		
AZT	azidothymidine (zidovudine)	CPR	cardiopulmonary resuscitation
BAL	British antilewisite (dimercaprol)	CREST	calcinosis, Raynaud's phenomenon, esophageal involvement, sclerodactyly, telangiectasia (syndrome)
BCG	bacille Calmette-Guérin		
BE	barium enema		
BP	blood pressure		

CRP	C-reactive protein	EMG	electromyography
CSF	cerebrospinal fluid	ENT	ears, nose, and throat
CSOM	chronic suppurative otitis media	EPVE	early prosthetic valve endocarditis
CT	cardiac transplant, computed tomography	ER	emergency room
		ERCP	endoscopic retrograde cholangiopancreatography
CVA	cerebrovascular accident		
CXR	chest x-ray	ERT	estrogen replacement therapy
d4T	didehydrodeoxythymidine (stavudine)	ESR	erythrocyte sedimentation rate
		ETEC	enterotoxigenic *E. coli*
DCS	decompression sickness	EtOH	ethanol
DDH	developmental dysplasia of the hip	FAP	familial adenomatous polyposis
		FEV_1	forced expiratory volume in 1 second
ddI	dideoxyinosine (didanosine)		
DES	diethylstilbestrol	FH	familial hypercholesterolemia
DEXA	dual-energy x-ray absorptiometry	FNA	fine-needle aspiration
DHEAS	dehydroepiandrosterone sulfate	FSH	follicle-stimulating hormone
DIC	disseminated intravascular coagulation	FTA-ABS	fluorescent treponemal antibody absorption test
DIF	direct immunofluorescence	FVC	forced vital capacity
DIP	distal interphalangeal (joint)	G6PD	glucose-6-phosphate dehydrogenase
DKA	diabetic ketoacidosis		
DL_{CO}	diffusing capacity of carbon monoxide	GABA	gamma-aminobutyric acid
		GERD	gastroesophageal reflux disease
DMSA	2,3-dimercaptosuccinic acid	GFR	glomerular filtration rate
DNA	deoxyribonucleic acid	GGT	gamma-glutamyltransferase
DNase	deoxyribonuclease	GH	growth hormone
2,3-DPG	2,3-diphosphoglycerate	GI	gastrointestinal
dsDNA	double-stranded DNA	GnRH	gonadotropin-releasing hormone
DSM	Diagnostic and Statistical Manual	GU	genitourinary
dsRNA	double-stranded RNA	GVHD	graft-versus-host disease
DTP	diphtheria, tetanus, pertussis (vaccine)	HAART	highly active antiretroviral therapy
		HAV	hepatitis A virus
DTPA	diethylenetriamine-penta-acetic acid	Hb	hemoglobin
		HbA-1C	hemoglobin A-1C
DTs	delirium tremens	HBsAg	hepatitis B surface antigen
DVT	deep venous thrombosis	HBV	hepatitis B virus
EBV	Epstein-Barr virus	hCG	human chorionic gonadotropin
ECG	electrocardiography	HCO_3	bicarbonate
Echo	echocardiography	Hct	hematocrit
ECM	erythema chronicum migrans	HCV	hepatitis C virus
ECT	electroconvulsive therapy	HDL	high-density lipoprotein
EEG	electroencephalography	HDL-C	high-density lipoprotein-cholesterol
EF	ejection fraction, elongation factor		
		HEENT	head, eyes, ears, nose, and throat (exam)
EGD	esophagogastroduodenoscopy		
EHEC	enterohemorrhagic *E. coli*	HELLP	hemolysis, elevated LFTs, low platelets (syndrome)
EIA	enzyme immunoassay		
ELISA	enzyme-linked immunosorbent assay	HFMD	hand, foot, and mouth disease
		HGPRT	hypoxanthine-guanine phosphoribosyltransferase
EM	electron microscopy		

5-HIAA	5-hydroxyindoleacetic acid	LFTs	liver function tests
HIDA	hepato-iminodiacetic acid (scan)	LH	luteinizing hormone
HIV	human immunodeficiency virus	LMN	lower motor neuron
HLA	human leukocyte antigen	LP	lumbar puncture
HMG-CoA	hydroxymethylglutaryl-coenzyme A	LPVE	late prosthetic valve endocarditis
		L/S	lecithin-sphingomyelin (ratio)
HMP	hexose monophosphate	LSD	lysergic acid diethylamide
HPI	history of present illness	LT	labile toxin
HPV	human papillomavirus	LV	left ventricular
HR	heart rate	LVH	left ventricular hypertrophy
HRIG	human rabies immune globulin	Lytes	electrolytes
HRS	hepatorenal syndrome	Mammo	mammography
HRT	hormone replacement therapy	MAO	monoamine oxidase (inhibitor)
HSG	hysterosalpingography	MCP	metacarpophalangeal (joint)
HSV	herpes simplex virus	MCTD	mixed connective tissue disorder
HTLV	human T-cell leukemia virus	MCV	mean corpuscular volume
HUS	hemolytic-uremic syndrome	MEN	multiple endocrine neoplasia
HVA	homovanillic acid	MI	myocardial infarction
ICP	intracranial pressure	MIBG	meta-iodobenzylguanidine (radioisotope)
ICU	intensive care unit		
ID/CC	identification and chief complaint	MMR	measles, mumps, rubella (vaccine)
IDDM	insulin-dependent diabetes mellitus		
		MPGN	membranoproliferative glomeru-lonephritis
IFA	immunofluorescent antibody		
Ig	immunoglobulin	MPS	mucopolysaccharide
IGF	insulin-like growth factor	MPTP	1-methyl-4-phenyl-tetrahy-dropyridine
IHSS	idiopathic hypertrophic subaortic stenosis		
		MR	magnetic resonance (imaging)
IM	intramuscular	mRNA	messenger ribonucleic acid
IMA	inferior mesenteric artery	MRSA	methicillin-resistant *S. aureus*
INH	isoniazid	MTP	metatarsophalangeal (joint)
INR	International Normalized Ratio	NAD	nicotinamide adenine dinucleotide
IP_3	inositol 1,4,5-triphosphate		
IPF	idiopathic pulmonary fibrosis	NADP	nicotinamide adenine dinu-cleotide phosphate
ITP	idiopathic thrombocytopenic purpura		
		NADPH	reduced nicotinamide adenine dinucleotide phosphate
IUD	intrauterine device		
IV	intravenous	NF	neurofibromatosis
IVC	inferior vena cava	NIDDM	non-insulin-dependent diabetes mellitus
IVIG	intravenous immunoglobulin		
IVP	intravenous pyelography	NNRTI	non-nucleoside reverse transcriptase inhibitor
JRA	juvenile rheumatoid arthritis		
JVP	jugular venous pressure	NO	nitric oxide
KOH	potassium hydroxide	NPO	nil per os (nothing by mouth)
KUB	kidney, ureter, bladder	NSAID	nonsteroidal anti-inflammatory drug
LCM	lymphocytic choriomeningitis		
LDH	lactate dehydrogenase	Nuc	nuclear medicine
LDL	low-density lipoprotein	NYHA	New York Heart Association
LE	lupus erythematosus (cell)	OB	obstetric
LES	lower esophageal sphincter	OCD	obsessive-compulsive disorder

OCPs	oral contraceptive pills	PTH	parathyroid hormone
OR	operating room	PTSD	post-traumatic stress disorder
PA	posteroanterior	PTT	partial thromboplastin time
PABA	para-aminobenzoic acid	PUVA	psoralen ultraviolet A
PAN	polyarteritis nodosa	PVC	premature ventricular contraction
P-ANCA	perinuclear antineutrophil cytoplasmic antibody	RA	rheumatoid arthritis
		RAIU	radioactive iodine uptake
Pao_2	partial pressure of oxygen in arterial blood	RAST	radioallergosorbent test
		RBC	red blood cell
PAS	periodic acid Schiff	REM	rapid eye movement
PAT	paroxysmal atrial tachycardia	RES	reticuloendothelial system
PBS	peripheral blood smear	RFFIT	rapid fluorescent focus inhibition test
Pco_2	partial pressure of carbon dioxide		
PCOM	posterior communicating (artery)	RFTs	renal function tests
		RHD	rheumatic heart disease
PCOS	polycystic ovarian syndrome	RNA	ribonucleic acid
PCP	phencyclidine	RNP	ribonucleoprotein
PCR	polymerase chain reaction	RPR	rapid plasma reagin
PCT	porphyria cutanea tarda	RR	respiratory rate
PCTA	percutaneous coronary transluminal angioplasty	RSV	respiratory syncytial virus
		RUQ	right upper quadrant
PCV	polycythemia vera	RV	residual volume
PDA	patent ductus arteriosus	Sao_2	oxygen saturation in arterial blood
PDGF	platelet-derived growth factor		
PE	physical exam	SBFT	small bowel follow-through
PEFR	peak expiratory flow rate	SCC	squamous cell carcinoma
PEG	polyethylene glycol	SCID	severe combined immunodeficiency
PEPCK	phosphoenolpyruvate carboxykinase		
		SERM	selective estrogen receptor modulator
PET	positron emission tomography		
PFTs	pulmonary function tests	SGOT	serum glutamic-oxaloacetic transaminase
PID	pelvic inflammatory disease		
PIP	proximal interphalangeal (joint)	SIADH	syndrome of inappropriate antidiuretic hormone
PKU	phenylketonuria		
PMDD	premenstrual dysphoric disorder	SIDS	sudden infant death syndrome
PML	progressive multifocal leukoencephalopathy	SLE	systemic lupus erythematosus
		SMA	superior mesenteric artery
PMN	polymorphonuclear (leukocyte)	SSPE	subacute sclerosing panencephalitis
PNET	primitive neuroectodermal tumor		
PNH	paroxysmal nocturnal hemoglobinuria	SSRI	selective serotonin reuptake inhibitor
Po_2	partial pressure of oxygen	ST	stable toxin
PPD	purified protein derivative (of tuberculosis)	STD	sexually transmitted disease
		T2W	T2-weighted (MRI)
PPH	primary postpartum hemorrhage	T_3	triiodothyronine
PRA	panel reactive antibody	T_4	thyroxine
PROM	premature rupture of membranes	TAH-BSO	total abdominal hysterectomy–bilateral salpingo-oophorectomy
PSA	prostate-specific antigen		
PSS	progressive systemic sclerosis		
PT	prothrombin time	TB	tuberculosis

TCA	tricyclic antidepressant	UPPP	uvulopalatopharyngoplasty
TCC	transitional cell carcinoma	URI	upper respiratory infection
TDT	terminal deoxytransferase	US	ultrasound
TFTs	thyroid function tests	UTI	urinary tract infection
TGF	transforming growth factor	UV	ultraviolet
THC	tetrahydrocannabinol	VDRL	Venereal Disease Research
TIA	transient ischemic attack		Laboratory
TLC	total lung capacity	VIN	vulvar intraepithelial neoplasia
TMP-SMX	trimethoprim-sulfamethoxazole	VIP	vasoactive intestinal polypeptide
tPA	tissue plasminogen activator	VLDL	very low density lipoprotein
TP-HA	*Treponema pallidum*	VMA	vanillylmandelic acid
	hemagglutination assay	V/Q	ventilation/perfusion (ratio)
TPP	thiamine pyrophosphate	VRE	vancomycin-resistant
TRAP	tartrate-resistant acid		enterococcus
	phosphatase	VS	vital signs
tRNA	transfer ribonucleic acid	VSD	ventricular septal defect
TSH	thyroid-stimulating hormone	vWF	von Willebrand's factor
TSS	toxic shock syndrome	VZV	varicella-zoster virus
TTP	thrombotic thrombocytopenic	WAGR	Wilms' tumor, aniridia,
	purpura		genitourinary abnormalities,
TURP	transurethral resection of the		mental retardation (syndrome)
	prostate	WBC	white blood cell
TXA	thromboxane A	WHI	Women's Health Initiative
UA	urinalysis	WPW	Wolff-Parkinson-White syndrome
UDCA	ursodeoxycholic acid	XR	x-ray
UGI	upper GI	ZN	Ziehl-Neelsen (stain)

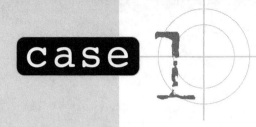

case 1

ID/CC   A **28-year-old** white male complains of severe **retrosternal pain** radiating to his left arm and jaw.

HPI   He has not had a physical exam as an adult. He adds that his **father died at a young age of a myocardial infarction.**

PE   Anguished, dyspneic, diaphoretic male with hand clutched to chest; soft, **elevated plaques on eyelids** (XANTHELASMAS); arcus senilis; painful **xanthomas of Achilles tendons** and patellae.

Labs   Elevated CK-MB; elevated troponin T and I. ECG: MI. **Extremely high LDL** cholesterol (650 mg/dL); **normal triglycerides** and **HDL.**

Imaging   Angio: coronary artery disease.

Gross Pathology   **Premature atherosclerosis** in large arteries.

Micro Pathology   Foam cells with lipid characteristic of atherosclerotic plaques.

case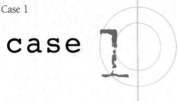

Familial Hypercholesterolemia

Differential

Type III Hyperlipidemia

Familial Defective apoB-100

Discussion

Familial hypercholesterolemia is also called **type II hyperlipoproteinemia**; it is an **autosomal-dominant defect in LDL receptor** with a gene frequency of 1:500. Homozygotes may have an eight-fold elevated LDL.

Treatment

Acute management of coronary artery disease; treatment of hyperlipidemia with dietary restriction, exercise, and cholesterol-lowering drugs, preferably **statins that are HMG-CoA reductase inhibitors** (simvastatin, atorvastatin, or rosuvastatin), and another LDL lowering drug such as niacin. Consider liver transplantation, LDL apheresis, or portocaval anastomosis in homozygous familial hypercholesterolemia.

Breakout Point

> ### LDL Receptor Mutant Classes:
> 1. Nulls with NO expression of LDL receptor
> 2. Defective transport from endoplasmic reticulum to Golgi = misfolding
> 3. Defective LDL binding to receptor (may affect VLDL)
> 4. Defective internalization to clathrin coated pits
> 5. Defective receptor recycling by inhibiting ligand-receptor dissociation

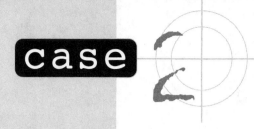

ID/CC A 16-year-old obese white male complains of sudden **midepigastric pain and nausea** after eating french fries.

HPI His history reveals that **he and a sibling** have had similar episodes of abdominal pain in the past. Careful questioning discloses that he experiences **flushing** every time he **drinks alcohol**.

PE **Nonpainful, yellowish papules on face, scalp, elbows, knees, and buttocks** (ERUPTIVE XANTHOMATOSIS); lipemia retinalis on funduscopic exam; hepatosplenomegaly; abdominal muscle guarding and palpable tenderness.

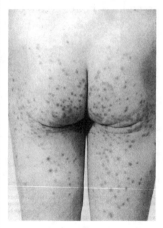

Figure 2-1. Eruptive xanthomas on the buttocks.

Labs **Elevated serum amylase** and lipase; **very high triglycerides (TGs)** >900 mg/dL; moderate elevation of serum cholesterol and phospholipids.

Micro Pathology Lipid-laden foam cells.

case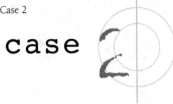

Familial Hypertriglyceridemia

Differential
Dysbetalipoproteinemia (Type III)

Acute Pancreatitis

Discussion
Familial hypertriglyceridemia is an autosomal-dominant common disorder in the United States, exacerbated by obesity and diabetes mellitus. Abdominal pain stems from **recurrent acute pancreatitis**. TGs are synthesized in the liver and intestine and packaged into lipoproteins that transport TGs and cholesterol via the circulation. Chylomicrons are made in liver; VLDL in the intestines.

Treatment
Low-fat diet; avoidance of alcohol; exercise; **fibric acid** and **niacin** in selected cases.

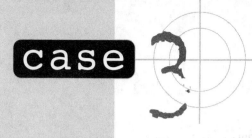

case

ID/CC A 54-year-old obese male is rushed to the ER after he was found **unconscious** on the floor of his office.

HPI He is taking medication for coronary artery disease.

PE On admission, he is found to be in an acute state of tissue **hypoperfusion** (SHOCK) with a barely palpable pulse, hypothermia, and bradycardia. Immediate treatment for cardiac shock is begun.

Labs ECG: acute anteroseptal myocardial infarction. **Increased serum lactate;** hyperphosphatemia. ABGs: **severe metabolic acidosis** (pH 7.27); bicarbonate 14 mEq/L (low). **Increased anion gap** (19) with no ketoacids; BUN and creatinine normal.

case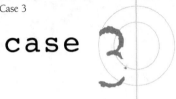

Lactic Acidosis

Differential Metabolic Acidosis
Cardiopulmonary Failure
Liver Failure
Alcoholic Ketoacidosis.

Discussion A state of increased levels of lactic acid in blood (LACTIC ACIDOSIS) may be due to a number of causes, including **shock** and **sepsis** (both increase lactic acid production due to hypoxia) or **circulatory failure**, methanol poisoning, metformin toxicity, and liver failure (failure of lactate removal from blood by its transformation to glucose). The anion gap is an estimation of the total unmeasured plasma anions, such as proteins, organic acids, phosphate, and sulfate. Increased anion-gap metabolic acidosis is due to salicylate poisoning, alcohol (e.g., methanol, ethanol, and propylene glycol) intoxication, lactic acidosis, renal failure, and diabetic ketoacidosis. L-lactate is only produced in humans with an excess due to increased anaerobic metabolism (hypoperfusion). D-lactate is produced by bacteria and present in patients with gastric bypass, small bowel resection, or short-gut syndrome.

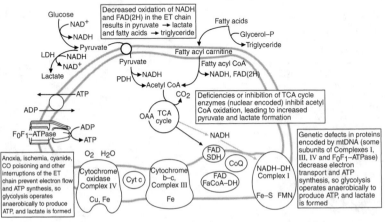

Figure 3-1. Pathways leading to lactic acidemia.

Treatment Treat precipitating cause of acidosis; administer alkalizing agents such as sodium bicarbonate if pH is <7.1. Treat shock.

case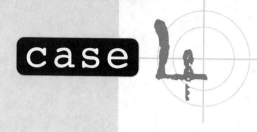

ID/CC A 34-year-old **farmer,** who returned from **military** service in the Middle East, is brought to the emergency room with **severe abdominal cramps** and **vomiting.**

HPI The patient is also **restless** and is **salivating profusely.** He has been excessively spraying a **pesticide** to prevent an insect outbreak.

PE Patient is nearly **stuporous; cyanosis** with marked respiratory distress; **bilateral miotic pupils; marked salivation** and **lacrimation;** moderate dehydration; **hyperactive bowel sounds; fecal and urinary incontinence.**

Labs ABGs: marked **hypoxemia** with **hypercapnia;** uncompensated **respiratory acidosis. Prerenal azotemia** on RFTs. Lytes: **hyperkalemia.**

Imaging CXR is normal.

case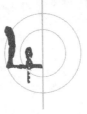

Pesticide (Organophosphate) Poisoning

Differential

Acute Respiratory Distress Syndrome
Chemical/Biological Warfare Agents
Congestive Heart Failure
Pulmonary Edema
Septic Shock
Asthma

Discussion

Organophosphates like parathion are widely used as pesticides, and several nerve agents developed for chemical warfare are rapid-acting and potent organophosphates. These agents act acutely and all of these toxins **inhibit the enzyme acetylcholinesterase,** inhibiting normal acetylcholine breakdown at cholinergic synapses. **Organophosphates cause irreversible inhibition,** but "ages" acetylcholinesterase, so with time, forms covalent bonds permanently disabling the enzyme.

Treatment

Specific therapy includes immediate administration of **atropine** (to offset cholinergic effects) and early initiation of **pralidoxime (PAM)** (chemically restores acetylcholinesterase if administered early to displace the organophosphate); supportive management for respiratory support and hemodialysis.

Breakout Point

DUMBELS Mnemonic—For Organophosphate Poisoning
D = Diarrhea and diaphoresis
U = Urination
M = Miosis
B = Bronchorrhea, bronchospasm, and brady-cardia
E = Emesis
L = Lacrimation
S = Salivation

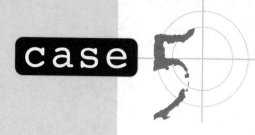

case 5

ID/CC   A 2-year-old girl, the daughter of a recently immigrated African family, is admitted to the pediatric ward owing to an **increase in abdominal girth** and **failure to thrive**.

HPI   She recently arrived in the United States from her home country. She was breast-fed until 1 year of age, at which time her mother ran out of milk. She is apathetic and irritable and has been having frequent episodes of diarrhea.

PE   **Height and weight in fifth percentile; skin and hair depigmentation;** thinning of hair; dry skin; hyperkeratosis on axillae and groin; hepatomegaly and **ascites;** generalized pitting **edema;** loss of muscle; lethargy.

Labs   CBC: anemia; lymphopenia. **Hypoalbuminemia** (normal in marasmus), **hypoproteinemia** and **hypoglycemia.** Lytes: hypokalemia; hypomagnesemia.

Imaging   US/CT: fatty liver. XR: delayed bone age.

Gross Pathology   **Fatty** infiltration of **liver.**

Micro Pathology   Intestinal mucosal atrophy with loss of brush border enzymes; atrophy of pancreatic islet cells; widespread fatty infiltration of liver.

NUTRITION

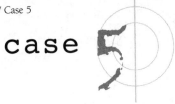

case 5

Kwashiorkor

Differential	Marasmus
	Actinic Prurigo
	Riboflavin Deficiency
Discussion	Kwashiorkor is a form of malnutrition caused by **protein deprivation** with **normal total caloric intake**.
Treatment	Restore acid-base and electrolyte balance; treat infections; gradually initiate high-protein diet with vitamins and minerals.

■ **TABLE 5-1 DIFFERENTIATING BETWEEN MILD AND SEVERE MALNUTRITION**

Extent of malnutrition	Moderate	Severe (Kwashiorkor)
Symmetric edema	No	YES
Height for given age	<2 S.D.	<3 S.D. (very stunted)
Weight:Height ratio	<2 S.D.	<3 S.D. (extreme wasting)

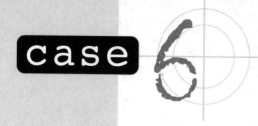

case 6

ID/CC An **18-month-old inner-city** boy is brought to the pediatric clinic by his parents because of **delayed dentition, poor growth and development,** frequent crying, and weakness.

HPI The infant's subsistence on breast milk with a **diet is deficient in** eggs, fish and **dairy products,** and he spends most of his time indoors (i.e., he has little **exposure to sunlight**).

PE **Softening of occipital and parietal bones with elastic recoil** (CRANIOTABES); frontal bossing; enlargement **of costochondral junctions** (RACHITIC ROSARY); **bowing of legs; lineal chest depression along diaphragm** (HARRISON'S GROOVE).

Labs **Serum calcium normal or slightly low; decreased serum phosphorus;** increased alkaline phosphatase; low 1,25$(OH)_2$-vitamin D level.

Imaging XR: **widening of growth plates;** osteopenia of cranial and long bones.

Gross Pathology Excess amount of **uncalcified bone** at junction of cartilage.

Micro Pathology Defective mineralization of osteoid in epiphysis and diaphysis.

NUTRITION

case 6

Rickets

Differential Bone Metastases

Discussion Rickets is a disease of infancy and childhood involving **defective mineralization of osteoid** in bone skeleton and the neuromuscular system because of **low vitamin D** or less commonly, low calcium or phosphorus in the diet; it can also be due to low sunlight exposure (vitamin D conversion in skin) and chronic renal failure (BUN and phosphorus levels are high).

Treatment Ultraviolet light exposure and vitamin D (cholecalciferol-vitamin D3) supplementation. May require calcium supplementation.

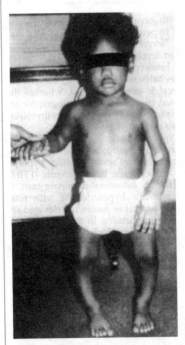

Figure 6-1. Nutritional rickets (vitamin D deficiency) in a 3-year-old boy. Note the severe bowing of the lower extremities and the widened wrists and ankles.

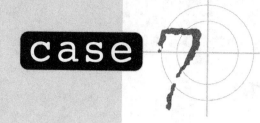

case 7

ID/CC	A 29-year-old Nepalese political dissident visits a medical clinic and is complaining of **diminished visual acuity, primarily at night.**
HPI	He recently arrived in the United States by boat after spending several years in a refugee camp.
PE	VS: normal. PE: conjunctiva shows diminished tear lubrication with dryness (XEROSIS; when localized, it forms patches known as Bitot's spots) as well as keratinization and small corneal ulcers (XEROPHTHALMIA).
Micro Pathology	Keratinizing metaplasia in conjunctiva; follicular hyperkeratosis with glandular plugging.

NUTRITION

case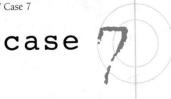

Vitamin A Deficiency

Differential | Keratosis

Discussion | Vitamin A (RETINOL) is a fat-soluble vitamin derived from beta-carotenes used for the **synthesis of rhodopsin** in the retina, for wound healing, and for epithelial cell growth and differentiation. Night blindness (NYCTALOPIA) is an early symptom of vitamin A deficiency; conjunctival xerosis and Bitot's spots are early signs. Corneal ulcers may progress to erosions and eventual destruction of cornea (KERATOMALACIA). Vitamin A deficiency can also result from alcoholism and malnutrition.

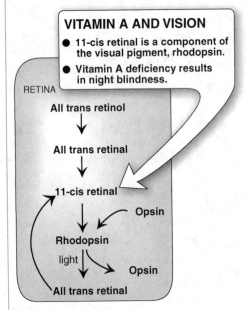

Figure 7-1. The role of vitamin A and vision.

Treatment | Vitamin A supplementation.

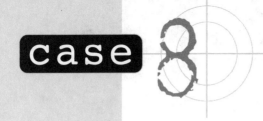

ID/CC   A 26-year-old white female comes to the family medicine clinic to have her 5-year-old daughter seen by a dermatologist because of **itching and scaling of her skin.**

HPI   The mother is very thin and fears that her daughter will not gain enough weight, so she has given her **cod-liver oil four times a day for the past nine months.** The child complains of **fatigue, headaches,** and **bone pain.**

PE   Funduscopic exam reveals **papilledema;** localized areas of hair loss (ALOPECIA); very **dry skin** with **scaling** areas on back and extremities; **hyperkeratosis** on medial side of soles of feet; **liver** moderately **enlarged** but not painful.

Imaging   XR, long bones and spine: **cortical hyperostosis; demineralization; premature closure of epiphyses.**

NUTRITION

case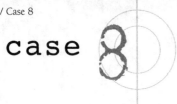

Vitamin A Toxicity

Differential | Exfoliative Dermatitis
Leukopenia
Pseudotumor Cerebri

Discussion | Together with vitamins D, E, and K, vitamin A is one of the **fat-soluble** vitamins, which means that the **body stores** them and does not eliminate them as quickly as it does water-soluble vitamins. Vitamin A (RETINOL) is derived from carotenes and is a constituent of retinal pigments (RHODOPSIN). Vitamin A is necessary for the integrity of all epithelial cells. **Deficiency of vitamin A** produces **night blindness** and **xerophthalmia.** Vitamin A is mainly found in meat, liver, fish, and dairy products. Hypervitaminosis A can cause congenital malformations in a developing fetus by excessive gene activation. Derivatives are teratogenic

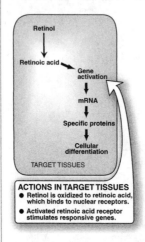

Figure 8-1. Vitamin A and cellular differentiation.

Treatment | Discontinue administration of vitamin A-containing supplement.

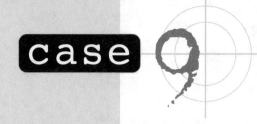

case 9

ID/CC A 39-year-old white male who is an **alcoholic** is brought to the emergency room with shortness of breath, confusion, **foot drop,** and swelling of his legs.

HPI He admits to getting drunk at least five times a week. His **diet** consists mainly of canned soup and cheap "junk food" high in carbohydrates and saturated fats when not binge drinking. He also complains of diarrhea.

PE VS: tachycardia. PE: dyspnea; jugular venous distention; **extremities warm** to touch; cardiomegaly; hepatomegaly; 2+ pitting edema of both lower extremities; confusion with **nystagmus;** decreased deep tendon reflexes.

Labs Low erythrocyte transketolase activity that increases <16% with administration of pyrophosphate is diagnostic; low serum and urine thiamine levels.

Imaging CXR: cardiomegaly with basal lung congestion.

Gross Pathology Wernicke encephalopathy shows congestion, hemorrhages, and necrosis in thalamus, hypothalamus **(mammillary bodies),** and paraventricular regions.

Micro Pathology Demyelinization of peripheral nerves with axonal degeneration and fragmentation.

case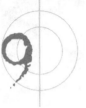

Vitamin B₁ Deficiency (Beriberi)

Differential

Alcoholism

Cirrhosis

Hyperthyroidism

Cardiomyopathy

Discussion

Lack of thiamine produces Wernicke-Korsakoff syndrome as well as **high-output heart failure (wet beriberi) and polyneuropathy (dry beriberi)**. Thiamine pyrophosphate (TPP) is a cofactor for the Krebs cycle enzymes α-ketoglutarate dehydrogenase and pyruvate dehydrogenase as well as transketolase (pentose phosphate pathway).

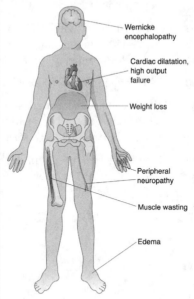

Figure 9-1. Complications of thiamine deficiency.

Treatment
Thiamine

Before administering glucose to an alcoholic, thiamine should be given to prevent encephalopathy (due to depletion of thiamine in glycolysis pathways). Alcoholics should also receive IV or oral folate and multivitamins.

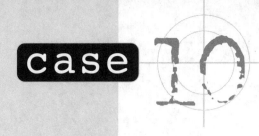

case 10

ID/CC   A 64-year-old **alcoholic** Hispanic female who recently underwent a strangulated hernia repair becomes weak, irritable with significant weight loss, and develops a **rash** on her face, neck, and the dorsum of her hands; she also suffers from **diarrhea** and **altered mental status.**

HPI   After her bowel resection, the patient became torpid and anorexic with lack of proper return of bowel function for one month. Her **diet** had been predominantly based on **corn** products.

PE   Erythematous, nonpruritic, hyperpigmented, scaling rash of face, neck (CASAL'S NECKLACE), and dorsum of hands; angular stomatitis (CHEILOSIS) and glossitis; diminished touch and pain sensation in all four extremities; apathy, confusion, and disorientation.

Labs   UA: low levels of urinary 2-pyridone and 2-methylnicotinamide are diagnostic.

Micro Pathology   Atrophy and ulceration of gastric and intestinal mucosa; posterior columns show neuronal degeneration and demyelination.

NUTRITION

case 10

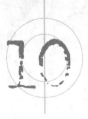

Pellagra

Differential

Atopic Dermatitis

Hartnup Disease

Lupus Erythematosus

Pemphigus

Porphyria Cutanea Tarda

Discussion

Pellagra is a final stage of Vitamin B$_3$ (NIACIN) deficiency (PELLAGRA) and is commonly seen in alcoholics and less frequently observed in patients with GI disorders or in elderly patients. GI tract problems precede dermatitis. In patients with carcinoid syndrome, tryptophan, the precursor of niacin, is used up to form serotonin. It is usually accompanied by other B vitamin deficiencies. Excessive corn consumption is a risk factor. The typical observed triad consists of **dermatitis, dementia, and diarrhea**, not necessarily in this order.

Breakout Point

Pellagra is manifested by the 4 Ds:
(photosensitive) **D**ermatitis **D**iarrhea **D**ementia **D**eath

Treatment

Oral nicotinamide.

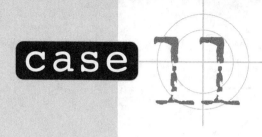

case 11

ID/CC A 10-month-old inner city white female is brought to the pediatric clinic because of **listlessness** and **anorexia**.

HPI She is the daughter of an unemployed, **poor** urban couple and has never before seen a pediatrician or taken any medication. Her parents report a diet of **unsupplemented, heated cow's milk**.

PE Weakness; pallor; **hyperkeratosis** and **hemorrhagic perifolliculitis** of skin of lower extremities, forearms, and abdomen; purpuric skin rashes; **splinter hemorrhages** in nail beds of hands; tenderness and swelling of distal femur and costochondral junctions; **bleeding gums; petechiae** seen over nasal and oral mucosa.

Labs CBC: microcytic, hypochromic anemia; leukopenia. Plasma and platelet levels of ascorbic acid low; **prolonged bleeding time**.

Imaging XR: subperiosteal hemorrhages; both legs and knees show "ground glass" appearance of bones and epiphyses.

Gross Pathology Growing bone shows diminished osteoid formation, hemarthrosis, and subperiosteal and periarticular hemorrhage; **defective collagen** (vitamin C hydroxylates proline and lysine); endochondral bone formation ceases (osteoblasts fail to form osteoid); existing trabeculae brittle and susceptible to fracture.

case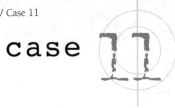

Vitamin C Deficiency (Scurvy)

Differential
Rheumatoid Arthritis
Child Abuse
Anemia
Acute Lymphoblastic Leukemia
Osteomyelitis
Rheumatic Fever

Discussion
Vitamin C (ASCORBIC ACID) deficiency, or scurvy, is observed in smokers, oncologic patients, alcoholics, infants, and the elderly resulting in **impaired collagen synthesis.**

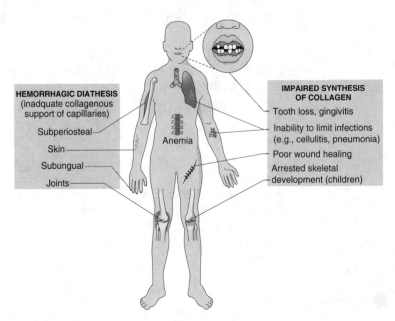

HEMORRHAGIC DIATHESIS
(inadquate collagenous support of capillaries)
Subperiosteal
Skin
Subungual
Joints

Anemia

IMPAIRED SYNTHESIS OF COLLAGEN
Tooth loss, gingivitis
Inability to limit infections (e.g., cellulitis, pneumonia)
Poor wound healing
Arrested skeletal development (children)

Figure 11-1. Complications of vitamin C deficiency (scurvy).

Treatment
Oral ascorbic acid (high doses may produce oxalate and uric acid stones).

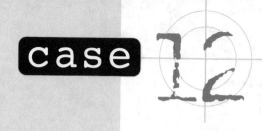

case 12

ID/CC A 47-year-old homeless **alcoholic** man (with a diet deficient in leafy vegetables) comes into the emergency room with weakness, **bleeding** gums, swelling in his right knee due to blood collection (HEMARTHROSIS), and **bloody vomit** (HEMATEMESIS).

HPI The patient's diet consists of one meal a day of leftovers from fast-food restaurants. He was **given ampicillin** for diarrhea **2 weeks ago** (leading to suppression of vitamin K synthesis by colonic bacteria).

PE Thin and **malnourished** with poor hygiene; conjunctival and nail bed pallor; **subcutaneous ecchymosis** in arms and legs; right knee **hemarthrosis**.

Labs Anemia (Hb 9.7); **prolonged PT and PTT**; normal platelet count, fibrinogen level, and thrombin time.

case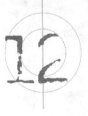

Vitamin K Deficiency

Differential	Leukemias
	Acute Lymphocytic Leukemia (ALL)
	Chronic Lymphocytic Leukemia (CLL)
	Chronic Myelogenous Leukemia (CML)
	Thrombocytopenic Purpura
	Scurvy (vitamin C deficiency)
Discussion	Coagulation factors II, VII, IX, and X are dependent on vitamin K for their activity (through gamma-carboxylation). Broad-spectrum antibiotic use, malabsorption, and lack of dietary vitamin K result in deficiency, manifested as bleeding. Clotting factors are synthesized in the liver; severe liver disease can cause coagulopathy.

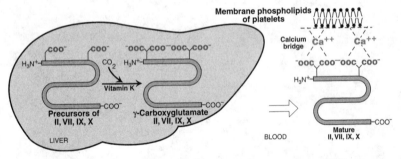

Figure 12-1. The role of vitamin K in blood coagulation.

Treatment	Vitamin K supplementation.

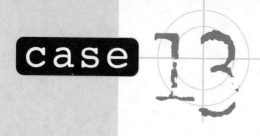

case

ID/CC   A newborn is evaluated by a pediatric endocrinologist because the intern performing the delivery **cannot discern whether the child is male or female** (AMBIGUOUS GENITALIA).

HPI   The child is also **lethargic** and lacks sufficient strength to suck on mother's milk adequately (due to salt wasting).

PE   Ambiguous external genitalia; **increase in size of clitoris; fusion of labia** to the point of resembling a scrotal sac.

Labs   Lytes: hyponatremia; **hyperkalemia. Increase in 17-α-OH progesterone** and its metabolite, **pregnanetriol; increase in urinary 17-ketosteroids** (defect is distal to 17, 20-desmolase); elevated serum ACTH. **Testosterone/dihydrotestosterone levels,** elevated ratio in serum. Prenatal diagnosis is possible at 14 to 16 weeks (due to increase in 17-α-OH progesterone). Karyotype: 46,XX female.

case 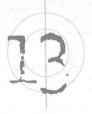 13

5-α-Reductase Deficiency

Differential

3-ß-Hydroxysteroid Dehydrogenase Deficiency

Ambiguous Genitalia

Androgen Insensitivity Syndrome

Discussion

Lack of 21-hydroxylase causes a decrease in cortisol with a consequent increase in ACTH, which in turn produces hyperplasia of the adrenals—resulting in an increase in androgen production that gives rise to signs of female pseudohermaphroditism (as in this case) or enlarged genitalia in the male. May occur with or without salt wasting. Bone mineralization should be monitored.

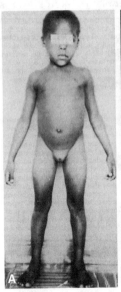 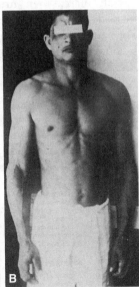

Figure 13-1. Two patients with 5α-reductase deficiencies. A, before puberty, the patient has a female phenotype. B, after puberty, a normal male body habitus develops.

Treatment

Cortisol; dehydrocorticosterone acetate if salt wasting is present; surgical correction of ambiguous genitalia; assigned female gender at birth.

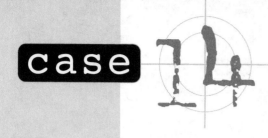

case

ID/CC A 16-year-old girl is referred to an endocrinologist owing to **lack of menses** (PRIMARY AMENORRHEA) and absence of pubic hair, axillary hair, and breast development (LACK OF SECONDARY SEXUAL CHARACTERISTICS).

HPI She also complains of frequent **headaches and ringing in her ears** (due to hypertension).

PE VS: **hypertension** (BP 160/105). PE: funduscopic exam normal; no lymphadenopathy; no hepatosplenomegaly; absence of breast tissue; no abdominal or pelvic masses palpable; no axillary or pubic hair; vulvar labia normal.

Labs Lytes: **hypokalemia;** hypernatremia. ABGs: metabolic **alkalosis** (due to mineralocorticoid action of 11-deoxycorticosterone and corticosterone). Suppressed renin; increase in urinary gonadotropins (due to attempt to compensate for lack of sex hormones); diminished 17-ketosteroids (product of sex hormones), serum estrogen; increased progesterone, pregnenolone, 11-deoxycorticosterone, and corticosterone.

ENDOCRINOLOGY

case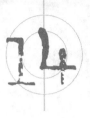

17-α-Hydroxylase Deficiency

Differential	5-Alpha Reductase Deficiency
	Hypogonadism
	Ambiguous Genitalia/Intersexuality
Discussion	An autosomal-recessive mutation of the **CYP17** gene leads to 17-α-hydroxylase deficiency. This deficiency leads in turn to impaired sex steroid and cortisol biosynthesis. Intermediary steroids have mineralocorticoid activity but no androgen activity. Excessive mineralocorticoid activity produces varying degrees of hypertension and hypokalemia. Thus, females fail to develop secondary sexual characteristics and males develop ambiguous external genitalia (MALE PSEUDO-HERMAPHRODITISM).

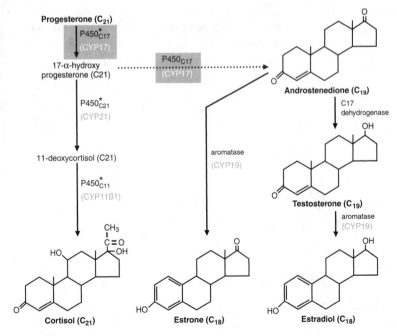

Figure 14-1. Mutation of the *CYP17* gene leads to 17-α-hydroxylase deficiency.

Treatment	Glucocorticoids. Sex hormones.

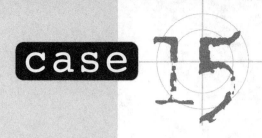

ID/CC A 41-year-old white male comes to the emergency room complaining of severe retro-orbital (behind his eyes) **headache** along with **blurred vision**.

HPI He also complains of weakness over the past few months and an **increase in hat size**. His family also notes a **coarsening of his facial features and deepening of his voice.**

PE VS: hypertension (BP 150/100). PE: skin thick and oily; **prominent forehead and jaw;** enlarged tongue and widening gaps between teeth; **large hands and feet; bitemporal hemianopsia; cardiomegaly;** hepatosplenomegaly.

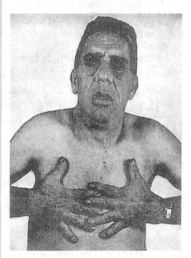

Figure 15-1. Patient at presentation.

Labs **Hyperglycemia;** hyperphosphatemia; **increased IGF-1; increased levels of GH** that **fail to suppress** after oral glucose load. UA: increased urinary calcium.

Imaging XR: thickening of skull; erosion and **enlargement of sella turcica.** MR, head: enlarged pituitary gland containing a 2-cm mass.

ENDOCRINOLOGY

29

case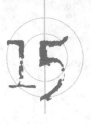

Acromegaly

Differential

Fragile X Syndrome

Marfan Syndrome

Hyperinsulinemia

Discussion

The most common cause (>95%) of acromegaly is a **GH-secreting pituitary adenoma.** If excess GH secretion is present in **childhood, gigantism** appears; **in adults, acromegaly** appears. Headache and joint pain are early complaints; blurred vision and visual-field changes occur later. Almost every organ in the body increases in size; 25% of patients exhibit glucose intolerance. Visual field changes (e.g., bitemporal hemianopsia) may occur secondary to compression of the nerves of the optic chiasm by the tumor.

Treatment

Transsphenoidal microsurgical adenomectomy is the first line therapy; radiotherapy to reduce further growth of tumor. Medical therapy with octreotide (a somatostain analogue, inhibits GH secretion and IGF-1) and/or bromocriptine (dopamine agonist, lowers serum GH) and/or pegvisomant (GH receptor antagonist) if surgery fails or is contraindicated.

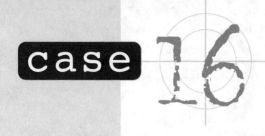
ID/CC A 40-year-old female is admitted to the medicine ward for evaluation of **increasing weakness** and intermittent episodes of **dizziness, nausea, and vomiting related to stress and exercise.** Symptoms have been occurring on and off for about a year.

HPI She is a vegetarian, takes no drugs or medications, and does not drink alcohol or smoke cigarettes. She reports an excessive **craving for salty foods** such as chips and salted peanuts.

PE VS: **tachycardia** (HR 110); **hypotension** (BP 90/65). PE: thin with dry mucous membranes; **pigmentation of buccal mucosa and palms of hands;** no neck masses; chest auscultation normal; no abdominal masses; no hepatosplenomegaly; no lymphadenopathy.

Labs CBC: normal. Lytes: **hyponatremia; hyperkalemia. Glucose low; increased BUN with normal creatinine;** amylase and LFTs normal; **high ACTH; low cortisol; rapid ACTH stimulation test** reveals failure of cortisol to rise above baseline.

Imaging CXR: indicates a smaller heart.

ENDOCRINOLOGY

case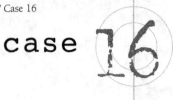

Addison Disease

Differential

Adrenal Crisis

C-17 Hydroxylase Deficiency

Adrenal Hemorrhage

Histoplasmosis

Sarcoidosis

Discussion

Primary hypoadrenalism (ADDISON DISEASE) may be caused by **idiopathic autoimmune mechanisms**, tuberculous infection, or sudden discontinuation of chronic steroid administration resulting in dysfunction of the entire adrenal cortex. Secondary hypoadrenalism is due to abnormalities of hypothalamic-pituitary function. Appearance in younger patients with **congenital adrenal hyperplasia.**

Treatment

Glucocorticoid and mineralocorticoid hormones. Hydrocortisone on an emergent basis for replacement therapy.

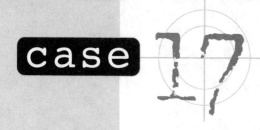
ID/CC After a routine pelvic exam, a 23-year-old **female** is referred by her family physician to an endocrinologist for an evaluation of "**lack of a palpable cervix.**"

HPI The patient states that she has **never had a menstrual period.**

PE **Bilateral breast tissue present; absence of pubic and axillary hair; vagina ends in blind pouch;** clitoromegaly; small atrophic **testis found** on right inguinal canal.

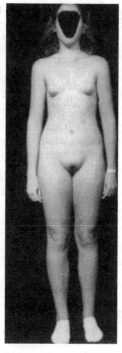

Figure 17-1. Patient on presentation.

Labs **Increased LH** and **testosterone.** Karyotype: **46,XY.**

Imaging US: uterus and ovaries absent.

33

case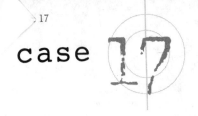

Androgen Insensitivity Syndrome

Differential 3-ß-Hydroxysteroid Dehydrogenase Deficiency
5-α Reductase Deficiency
17-α-Hydroxylase Deficiency

Discussion Also known as testicular feminization is an **X-linked recessive** condition characterized by a genotypically male individual (KARYOTYPE 46,XY) who presents with a female body habitus with breast development and cryptorchidism; it is due to a Y chromosome loss-of-function mutation in the androgen receptor gene that causes the **androgen receptor protein to be unresponsive to androgenic stimulation,** though there is normal testosterone to dihydrotestosterone conversion.

Treatment Treat on the basis of **gender identity preference.** Options include hormone replacement therapy with estrogens and psychological support. Surgery (orchidectomy) is an option depending on the gender preference. Resection of the cryptorchid testis and look for the intra-abdominal one (due to high risk of malignancy). Psychological morbidity is high for phenotypic females who are genotypic males.

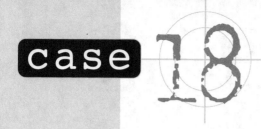

ID/CC A **15-year-old** female is admitted to the medicine ward for evaluation of persistent **weakness** for the last 6 months that has been unresponsive to multivitamin treatment.

HPI She denies allergies, surgeries, psychological problems, transfusions, drug use, or any relevant past medical history. She craves salt and is often constipated.

PE VS: heart rate normal; no fever; **normal BP** (excludes primary hyperaldosteronism). PE: short in stature, well hydrated; pupils equal and reactive to light and accommodation; no neck masses; no lymphadenopathy; chest normal; abdomen soft and nontender; no masses; neurologic exam normal; **no peripheral edema;** sexual development appropriate for age.

Labs CBC: normal. Lytes: **hyponatremia; severe hypokalemia.** ABGs: **metabolic alkalosis. Increased plasma renin** (excludes primary hyperaldosteronism); increased urinary excretion of prostaglandins. Magnesium is normal (excludes Gitelman's syndrome).

Micro Pathology **Juxtaglomerular cell hyperplasia** on renal biopsy.

ENDOCRINOLOGY

case 18

Bartter Syndrome

Differential

Hypokalemia

Metabolic Acidosis

Cystic Fibrosis

Discussion

Classic Bartter syndrome may be an autosomal recessive hereditary disorder characterized by a defective ClC-kb chloride channel in the thick ascending loop of Henle. Many cases are sporadic in nature. This results in an impaired mechanism of chloride to exit the cell and an inhibition of the potassium chloride/sodium chloride cotransporter with urinary sodium wasting and a consequent increase in renin production (through increased renal prostaglandins). Therefore, there is an increase in aldosterone activity with hypokalemic metabolic alkalosis in the absence of edema or hypertension. Hypokalemia perpetuates the cycle by stimulating renin activity.

Treatment

Indomethacin to decrease prostaglandin synthesis. Potassium chloride supplements and potassium-sparing diuretics.

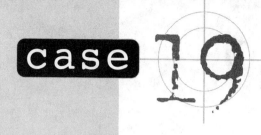

case 19

ID/CC A 26-year-old airline attendant is seen in the emergency room because of malaise, **confusion, abdominal pain,** vomiting, and diarrhea.

HPI She is a known **insulin-dependent diabetic** (IDDM type I, juvenile onset). The night before her admission, she went out to celebrate her birthday and drank excess **alcohol** until she became intoxicated (she also forgot to administer insulin).

PE VS: tachycardia (HR 92); hypotension (BP 90/50) (due to hypovolemia); **rapid, deep breathing** (KUSSMAUL RESPIRATION). PE: **dehydration;** peripheral cyanosis; cold, **dry skin; peculiar fruity breath smell** (due to ketone bodies, acetoacetate, and β-OH-butyrate).

Labs CBC: leukocytosis (14,000) (without infection). Lytes: hyponatremia (130 mEq/L). ABGs: **markedly reduced bicarbonate** (10 mEq/L); **acidosis** (pH <7.1). Increased ketones in blood; increased creatinine; **hyperglycemia; increased anion gap** (between 10 and 18) (anion gap is calculated as follows: $[Na + K] - [Cl + HCO_3]$). UA: glycosuria; ketonuria.

case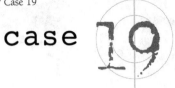

Diabetic Ketoacidosis

Differential

Metabolic Acidosis

Alcoholic Ketoacidosis

Hyperosmolar Coma

Discussion

Ketoacidosis involves hyperglycemia, acidosis, and ketosis and might be a first manifestation of diabetes. It is more common in an untreated insulin deficiency in insulin-dependent diabetics than hyperosmolar coma. It usually follows a period of physical or mental stress (e.g., MI, acute grief) or infection.

Breakout Point

The Four "I's" Causing Diabetic Ketoacidosis

Ischemia (myocardial infarction)

Insulinopenia (new onset or noncompliance)

Infection

Iatrogenic (steroids)

Treatment

IV fluid repletion; electrolyte management, especially potassium supplementation; parenteral insulin administration. Monitor with frequent measurement of blood glucose, serum ketones, arterial pH, and anion gap.

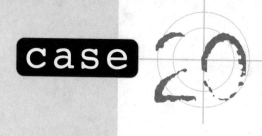

case

ID/CC A 27-year-old white male complains of **excessive thirst** (POLYDIPSIA) and **increased urination** (POLYURIA) with very diluted urine.

HPI The patient drinks several liters of water every day. He was well until this time. The patient also admits to frequent urination (including **nocturia**) of large volumes that are clear and watery.

PE VS: slight tachycardia. PE: mild dryness of mucous membranes; visual field testing normal; no papilledema; pupils equal and reactive.

Labs **Low urine specific gravity** (<1.006); **low urine osmolarity** (<200 mOsm/L); **elevated serum osmolality** (>290 mOsm/L); **hypernatremia; water deprivation test** demonstrates inability to concentrate urine with fluid restriction (urinary osmolality continues to be low).

Imaging CT: may show masses or lesions in hypothalamus.

case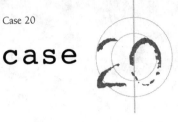

Diabetes Insipidus

Differential
Type I Diabetes (Mellitus)
Head Trauma
Histiocytosis X
Psychogenic Polydipsia
Osmotic Diuresis

Discussion
Diabetes insipidus is caused by an ADH deficiency (PRIMARY) or by renal unresponsiveness to ADH (NEPHROGENIC OR SECONDARY). Primary diabetes insipidus can be caused by surgical, traumatic, idiopathic (this case), or anoxic damage to the hypothalamus or pituitary stalk during pregnancy (SHEEHAN SYNDROME). Deficiency of ADH results in **renal loss of free water and hypernatremia.**

Treatment
Central (primary) diabetes insipidus: intranasal desmopressin and ADH-releasing drugs such as chlorpropamide, carbamazepine, and clofibrate. Nephrogenic (secondary) diabetes insipidus: add indomethacin, amiloride, and/or hydrochlorothiazide.

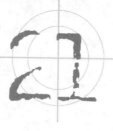
ID/CC   A 58-year-old white **female** comes to see her internist because of **weight loss**, the development of **polyuria, polydipsia** (due to hyperglycemia), and a **skin eruption** that comes and goes in different parts of her body

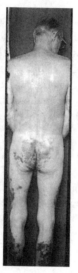

Figure 21-1. Necrolytic migratory erythema.

HPI   She also complains of increasing intermittent **diarrhea, nausea, vomiting, weight loss,** and occasional weakness and dizziness.

PE   VS: normal. PE: patient well hydrated; marked pallor; **erythematous rash on anterior chest, legs, and arms;** no neck masses; lungs clear to auscultation; heart sounds rhythmic; abdomen soft; no masses; no peritoneal signs; no lymphadenopathy.

Labs   CBC: anemia (Hb 7.4 mg/dL). **Markedly hyperglycemia.**

Imaging   MR/CT: 2.5-cm enhancing mass in body and tail of pancreas; several liver metastases.

ENDOCRINOLOGY

case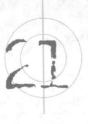

Glucagonoma

Differential

Type 1 Diabetes

Type 2 Diabetes

Mucocutaneous Candidiasis

Cirrhosis

Discussion

Glucagonoma is a pancreatic islet cell neoplasm that secretes abnormally high amounts of glucagon with resulting **symptomatic hyperglycemia**; it may also secrete gastrin, ACTH, and serotonin. Glucagonomas arise from alpha 2 islet cells in the pancreas, and the majority (>75%) are malignant. Glucagonomas may also be associated with multiple endocrine neoplasias (MEN) type I.

Treatment

Surgical removal. Streptozocin and doxorubicin if metastatic; insulin; prophylactic heparin and zinc (for skin rash); octreotide (somatostatin analogue inhibiting pituitary hormone secretion).

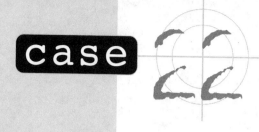
ID/CC   A 41-year-old woman is referred to an internist by her family practitioner because of persistent **hypertension** that has been **unresponsive to conventional treatment;** she also complains of profound **muscle weakness** (due to hypokalemia).

PE   VS: normal heart rate; **hypertension** (BP 200/100). PE: no pallor; **retinal hemorrhages, exudates, and AV nicking;** lungs clear; no heart murmurs; abdomen soft; no palpable masses; no lymphadenopathy.

Labs   CBC: increased hematocrit. Lytes: **hypokalemia; hypernatremia.** ABGs: metabolic alkalosis. Glucose normal (vs. ectopic ACTH production). ECG: left ventricular hypertrophy and strain. UA: no proteinuria. **Aldosterone levels high; renin levels low.**

Imaging   CT/MR: 1.7-cm enhancing left adrenal mass.

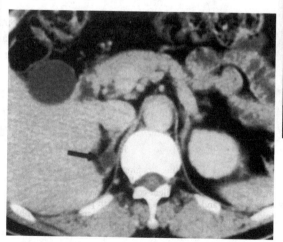

Figure 22-1. Relatively lucent focal areas of decreased attenuation suggestive of a mass (*arrow*).

ENDOCRINOLOGY

case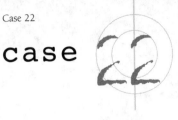

Hyperaldosteronism—Primary

Differential

Conn Syndrome

Cushing Syndrome

C-11 Hydroxylase Deficiency

C-17 Hydroxylase Deficiency

Discussion

Primary hyperaldosteronism is one of the most common causes of secondary hypertension and typically presents with hypertension, hypokalemia, hypernatremia, and increased bicarbonate due to increased secretion of aldosterone by an adrenal adenoma (CONN SYNDROME) or hyperplasia. Potential causes are aldosteronoma and idiopathic adrenal hyperplasia. Hypertension is characteristically **unresponsive to ACE inhibitors.** Surgically correctable causes of hypertension include Conn syndrome, pheochromocytoma, renal artery stenosis, and coarctation of the aorta.

Treatment

Surgical excision of adrenal mass; dietary sodium restriction and aldosterone antagonists such as spironolactone are also effective.

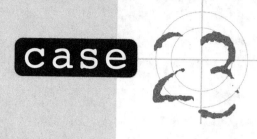

case 2

ID/CC   A 55-year-old menopausal female comes to see her internist because of progressive **constipation** and **excessive urination** over the past 2 months; she also complains of intermittent abdominal pain.

HPI   She has read "all about" osteoporosis during menopause and is afraid of developing it, so she has been taking **massive** amounts of **calcium supplements** and vitamin D injections.

PE   VS: hypertension; bradycardia. PE: lungs clear; no neck masses; thyroid not palpable; no lymphadenopathy; **muscle weakness with hyperreflexia;** abdomen soft with decreased bowel sounds; no masses; no abnormal pigmentation.

Labs   **Markedly increased serum calcium** (12 mg/dL) (always correct calcium level for serum albumin). Phosphorus normal (makes primary hyperparathyroidism less likely). ABGs: metabolic alkalosis. Increased BUN. ECG: **short Q-T.** No PTH-related protein detected.

case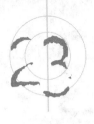

Hypercalcemia

Differential

Hyperparathyroidism
Hyperkalemia
Hyperphosphatemia
Hypernatremia
Hypermagnesemia

Discussion

Hypercalcemia may occur in hyperparathyroidism, milk-alkali syndrome, multiple myeloma, Addison disease, sarcoidosis, prolonged immobilization, metastatic neoplastic disease (due to increased osteoclastic resorption), and primary neoplastic disease (due to production of a PTH-like substance). Ninety-eight percent of the body's calcium is in the skeleton; 50% of the remaining serum calcium is bound to albumin. Free calcium is biologically active and is reabsorbed in the proximal tubule together with sodium. This reabsorption is decreased with expansion of extracellular fluid volume. The majority of cases of hypercalcemia are caused by hyperparathyroidism or bony metastases.

Breakout Point

Corrected calcium (mg/dL) = measured total Ca (mg/dL) + 0.8 (4.0 − serum albumin [g/dL]), where 4.0 represents the average albumin level.

Treatment

Aggressive rehydration with normal saline; diuresis with furosemide to increase sodium and concomitant calcium excretion. Calcitonin, gallium nitrate, or bisphosphonates (etidronate, pamidronate) may be necessary.

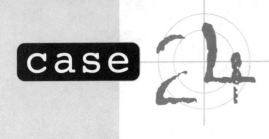

case 24

ID/CC	A 56-year-old Asian **female** goes to her family doctor for a routine physical and is found to be **hypercalcemic**.
HPI	She is asymptomatic except for mild **polyuria** and some **bone pain**.
PE	VS: mild **hypertension.** PE: no neck masses; thyroid not palpable; no lymphadenopathy; lungs clear; heart sounds normal; abdomen soft; no masses.
Labs	**Increased serum calcium; phosphorus low; elevated PTH; increased alkaline phosphatase**. UA: increased urinary calcium; elevated urinary cAMP and hydroxy-proline levels. ABGs: **hyperchloremic metabolic acidosis** (normal anion gap). ECG: **short Q-T.**
Imaging	XR: subperiosteal bone resorption; **cystic long-bone lesions** (BROWN TUMORS). Nuc: reduced cortical bone density in extremities and preserved spinal cancellous bone density. US: well defined hypoechoic lesion with necrosis.
Gross Pathology	Soft, round, well-encapsulated, yellowish-brown single parathyroid adenoma weighing 2 g.
Micro Pathology	Chief cells within adenoma.

ENDOCRINOLOGY

case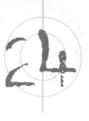

Hyperparathyroidism—Primary

Differential

Secondary Hyperparathyroidism

Hypercalcemia

Familial Benign (hypocalciuric) Hypercalcemia

Discussion

The parathyroid glands are primarily responsible for maintaining extracellular calcium concentrations via secretion of parathyroid hormone. Primary unregulated hypersecretion of parathyroid hormone may be caused by an **adenoma** (vast majority of cases), chief-cell hyperplasia, or carcinoma of the parathyroid glands; it is commonly asymptomatic and frequently recognized during routine physical exams. When it is symptomatic, peptic ulcer pain, polyuria, polydipsia, constipation, and pancreatitis may be the presenting symptoms. May be associated with multiple endocrine neoplasias (MEN) syndromes I and II.

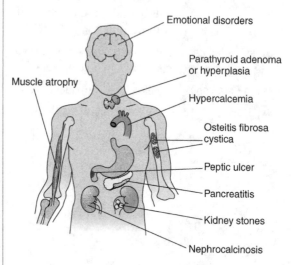

Figure 24-1. Major clinical features of hyperparathyroidism.

Treatment

Surgical removal.

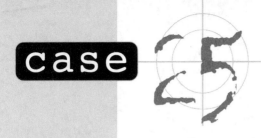

ID/CC A 32-year-old female visits her family doctor because of anxiety, palpitations, **intolerance to heat,** nervousness with **trembling hands,** and **weight loss** despite a normal appetite.

HPI She is also concerned about increasing **protrusion of her eyes** (EXOPHTHALMOS). Her grandmother had Hashimoto thyroiditis.

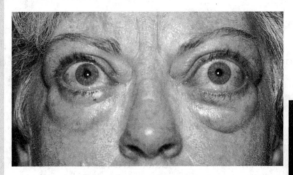

Figure 25-1. Exophthalmos.

PE VS: **tachycardia;** hypertension (BP 150/80). PE: wide pulse pressure; sweaty palms; warm skin; exophthalmos (due to enlargement of extraocular muscles); **generalized enlargement of thyroid gland** with bruit (DIFFUSE GOITER); nodular lesions over anterior aspect of lower legs (PRETIBIAL MYXEDEMA).

Labs **Markedly decreased TSH** (due to negative feedback of autonomously secreted thyroid hormones); **increased T_3, T_4, and free T_4 index;** positive thyroid-stimulating antibodies; positive antithyroglobulin and antiperoxidase antibodies; hypercalcemia. CBC: anemia.

Micro Pathology Thyroid gland hypertrophy and hyperplasia; reduced thyroid hormone storage and colloid; lymphoid infiltration of stroma; infiltrative ophthalmopathy.

ENDOCRINOLOGY

case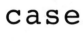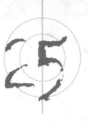

Hyperthyroidism (Graves Disease)

Differential

Subacute Thyroiditis
Pituitary Adenomas (thyroid-secreting)
Hashimoto Thyroiditis
Anxiety Disorder

Discussion

Also called diffuse toxic goiter (and Basedow disease in Europe); Graves disease is the most common cause of hyperthyroidism. It is idiopathic in nature but is an **autoimmune disease** mediated by **B-lymphocytes with thyrotropin receptor as the major autoantigen** and is associated with HLA on chromosome 6 and *CTLA4, HLA-DRB1*, and *HLA-DQB1*. Signs and symptoms are due to excess circulating thyroid hormone. Often patients have a **family history of autoimmune thyroid diseases.**

Treatment

Antithyroid drugs (propylthiouracil, methimazole); radioactive iodine; surgery if medical therapy fails. **Eye care for Graves opthalmopathy is essential.**

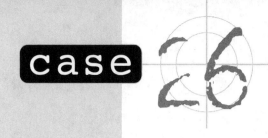

ID/CC　A 73-year-old female complains of **weakness, painful muscle cramps,** and **constipation.**

HPI　She suffers from chronic congestive heart failure (CHF) that has been treated with **digoxin** and **furosemide.** She was also on oral potassium tablets but has discontinued them because of gastric upset.

PE　VS: irregularly irregular pulse (atrial fibrillation); hypertension (BP 145/90); no fever. PE: well hydrated; conjunctiva normal; jugular venous pulse slightly increased, S3 heard; mild hepatomegaly and pitting edema of lower legs (all due to CHF); deep tendon **reflexes hypoactive.**

Labs　CBC: normal. Lytes: **Pending.**

ECG: flattening of S-T segment and T waves; **prominent U waves.**

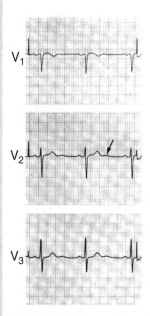

Figure 26-1. Note prominent U waves (*arrow*).

51

case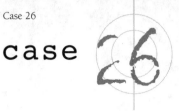

Hypokalemia

Differential

Cushing Syndrome

Hypocalcemia

Hypomagnesemia

Discussion

Potent diuretics such as furosemide frequently cause excessive renal loss of potassium with symptomatic hypokalemia which, if severe, may be life-threatening. **In patients on digoxin, hypokalemia greatly increases toxicity.** Potassium is the **most abundant intracellular action** in the body.

Treatment

Potassium-rich foods (chick peas, bananas, papaya); oral or parenteral potassium replacement; gastric mucosal protective agents; magnesium supplements (deficiency of magnesium frequently coexists). Potassium-sparing diuretics.

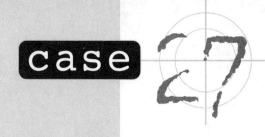

case 27

ID/CC   A 48-year-old female who has been **on total parenteral nutrition** for 2 weeks complains of **muscle weakness,** cramps, **palpitations, tremors, and depression.**

HPI   One week ago, she underwent her fifth major abdominal operation for intestinal fistula and sepsis.

PE   VS: **tachycardia;** hypotension. PE: patient looks **confused** and "run down"; agitation with muscular **spasticity and hyperreflexia;** heart sounds disclose skipped beats; mild hypoaeration at lung bases; abdomen with three colostomy bags at site of fistula; no peritoneal irritation; no surgical wound infection.

Labs   CBC: neutrophilic leukocytosis. Lytes: **Pending.** ECG: **prolonged P-R and Q-T intervals; wide QRS; tall T waves; premature ventricular ectopic contractions.**

case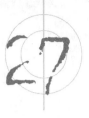

Hypomagnesemia

Differential

Hypokalemia

Hypocalcemia

Discussion

Homeostasis of magnesium is achieved through a balance between intestinal (small bowel) absorption and urinary excretion. Magnesium is the second most abundant intracellular cation in the body (after potassium). Deficiency is associated with the use of a large amount of IV fluids, alcoholism, intestinal malabsorption or diarrhea, inadequate replacement in parenteral nutrition, kwashiorkor or marasmus, prolonged GI losses such as suction, intestinal fistula, renal tubular acidosis, and use of drugs such as diuretics, cisplatin, methotrexate, amphotericin B, cyclosporine, and aminoglycosides.

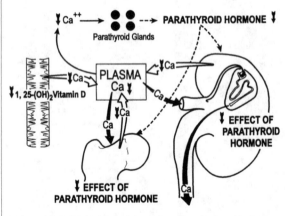

Figure 27-1. Disturbance of calcium metabolism during magnesium deficiency.

Treatment

Magnesium supplementation; magnesium sulfate if severe depletion. Hypokalemia and hypocalcemia resolve with magnesium replacement.

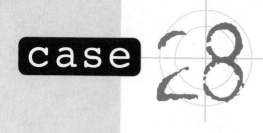

case 28

ID/CC A 33-year-old white female complains of **nausea, vomiting, and headache** on her first postoperative day; later, the charge nurse found her having a grand mal seizure.

HPI She had **elective surgery** for a benign left ovarian cyst. Her medical history discloses no previous illness.

PE VS: no fever; normal heart rate. PE: well hydrated; slight **confusion and lethargy** as well as general **weakness;** normal JVP; no bleeding or dehiscence (opening of surgical wound) or infection from surgical wound; no peritoneal signs; no lower extremity edema.

Labs CBC: normal. Lytes: hyponatremia (Na 115). Remainder of routine lab exams normal; normal cortisol (done to exclude possible adrenal insufficiency); serum osmolality <280.

ENDOCRINOLOGY

case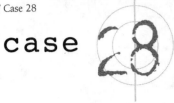

Hyponatremia

Differential

Renal Failure

Adrenal Crisis

Congestive Heart Failure

Syndrome of Inappropriate ADH Secretion

Discussion

Hyponatremia is the most common electrolyte disturbance seen in hospitalized patients and is often iatrogenic in nature. In a postoperative setting, the **metabolic response** to trauma is to **increase secretion of antidiuretic hormone** (ADH), among other hormones, which, coupled with overzealous IV administration of hypotonic fluids, may lead to symptomatic hyponatremia.

Treatment

For isovolemic hyponatremia (this case): free water restriction, discontinuation of hypotonic IV fluids. Severe symptomatic hyponatremia may require hypertonic (3%) saline therapy or antagonists to arginine vasopressin. For hypervolemic hyponatremia: fluid restriction, careful diuresis. Overly rapid correction of sodium concentration may lead to **central pontine myelinosis**, which is characterized by pseudobulbar palsy, spastic quadriparesis, dysarthria, and dysphagia.

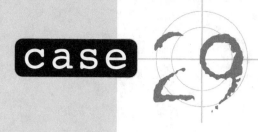

case 29

ID/CC   A 22-year-old woman is referred to the endocrinologist because of concern over **excessive facial hair** along with hair on her central chest and thighs.

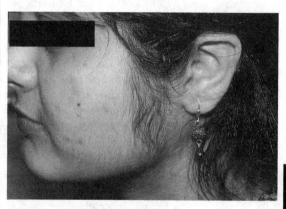

Figure 29-1. Excessive facial hair.

HPI   The patient's **menses are regular,** with an average flow lasting 3 to 4 days. She is not taking any drugs.

PE   Hirsutism noted; **no clitoromegaly** present (no evidence of virilization); no abdominal or pelvic mass palpable per abdomen or per vagina.

Labs   **Normal total testosterone** levels; **normal DHEAS;** normal urine for 17-ketosteroids.

Imaging   US: abdomen and pelvis: both adrenals and ovaries normal.

case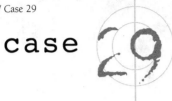

Hirsutism—Idiopathic

Differential

Adrenal Adenoma

Cushing Syndrome

C-11 Hydroxylase Deficiency

C-17 Hydroxylase Deficiency

Epidermolysis Bullosa

Discussion

Hirsutism that is disproportionate to the patient's ethnic background and is accompanied by normal periods is termed idiopathic. If testosterone (the major circulating androgen) and DHEAS (dehydroepiandrosterone sulfate, an adrenal cortical androgen) levels are normal, the patient can be reassured that the condition is benign. If the onset of hirsutism is pubertal with irregular periods, the possibility of polycystic ovarian syndrome exists. Recent onset hirsutism in an adult female, especially when associated with amenorrhea, requires complete investigation to exclude an adrenal or ovarian tumor.

Treatment

Cosmetic and/or dermatologic management including laser therapy; oral contraceptives inhibiting ovarian androgen production or flutamide (nonsteroidal antiandrogen) may be beneficial in selected cases.

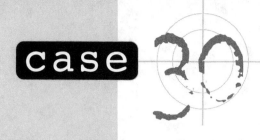

case

ID/CC   A 17-year-old white female student who is learning how to inject herself with **insulin** is found **unconscious** by her desk.

HPI   The patient suffered from weight loss, polyuria, polydipsia, and polyphagia for several months and was recently diagnosed with **juvenile-onset diabetes mellitus.** She has been meticulous in self-administering insulin injections.

PE   VS: **tachycardia** (HR 96); **hypotension** (BP 100/50); no fever. PE: **skin cold and moist;** patient **stuporous** with hyporeflexia; negative Babinski sign; responsive only to painful stimuli; cardiopulmonary exam normal; no hepatomegaly; no splenomegaly; no peritoneal signs.

Labs   **Severe hypoglycemia.** Lytes: potassium and magnesium levels sharply decreased (HYPOKALEMIA, HYPOMAGNESEMIA). BUN and creatinine normal; normal C-peptide levels.

Imaging   CT: head: no intracranial pathology demonstrated to account for the stuporous state.

case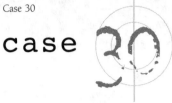

Insulin Overdose

Differential | Drug Overdose
Delirium

Discussion | With the administration of insulin, blood glucose levels are lowered by direct stimulation of cellular uptake. Glucose uptake is accompanied by a shift of magnesium and potassium into the cell. A severe hypoglycemic coma may result from an insulin overdose, which can produce **permanent neurologic damage or death.**

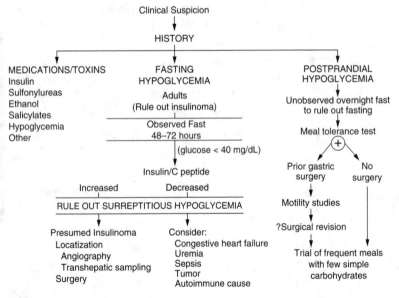

Figure 30-1. Algorithm for evaluation of hypoglycemia.

Treatment | Administer IV 50% glucose after drawing baseline blood sample. Follow serum glucose levels for several hours; monitor and treat electrolyte imbalances (potassium chloride).

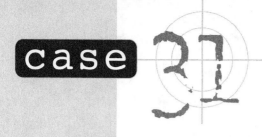
ID/CC A 53-year-old obese white female who works as a janitor is brought to the ER **in a coma** after being found on the floor of her room.

HPI Her husband reveals that she has been having **episodes of early morning dizziness, blurred vision,** and confusion associated with **hunger;** he adds that these **symptoms disappear after eating.** He also states that the patient has frequently been **nervous and irritable.**

PE VS: tachycardia (HR 105); BP normal. PE: patient comatose; mild skin pallor; **cold, sweaty hands.**

Labs Normal hemoglobin (14.4 mg/dL); BUN and creatinine normal. Lytes: normal. **Hypoglycemia; elevated plasma immunoreactive C-peptide.** Positive 72-hour fasting test.

Imaging CT: 1.5-cm **mass in tail of pancreas.** Nuc: mass takes up octreotide.

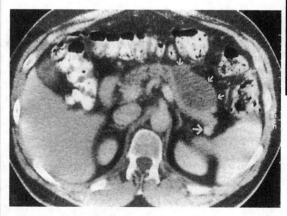

Figure 31-1. Pancreatic mass (arrows).

ENDOCRINOLOGY

case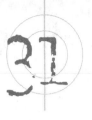

Insulinoma

Differential

Hypoglycemia
Surreptitious Insulin Administration
Lithium Toxicity
Hypothyroidism
Alcohol Intoxication

Discussion

The most common pancreatic endocrine tumor. Pancreatic islet cell tumor is beta-cell insulinoma (usually benign). Other types include glucagonomas, somatostatinomas, gastrinomas (ZOLLINGER-ELLISON SYNDROME), and excessive VIP-secreting tumor (VERNER-MORRISON SYNDROME). Islet cell tumors may be seen in multiple endocrine neoplasias (MEN) syndromes.

Treatment

Immediate IV glucose infusion for hypoglycemia; surgical resection.

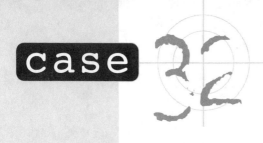

case 32

ID/CC	An 18-year-old male presents with lack of muscle strength and a high-pitched voice.
HPI	He has a **cleft lip and palate.** On directed questioning, he reports a **greatly diminished sense of smell** (HYPOSMIA). He also admits to a lack of libido and erectile dysfunction.
PE	VS: normal. PE: left cleft lip and incomplete unilateral cleft palate; marked **hyposmia** on olfactory testing; heart and lung sounds within normal limits; sparse facial and body hair; small penis and testes (prepubertal); **lack of scrotal pigmentation;** no palpable mass in abdomen and pelvis.

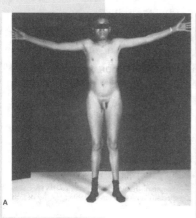
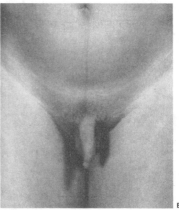

Figure 32-1. Patient on presentation.

Labs	CBC/Lytes: normal. LFTs normal; **decreased GnRH; low FSH and LH; low testosterone.**
Imaging	XR: skull: normal sella turcica. MR: brain: absent olfactory bulb(s).

ENDOCRINOLOGY

case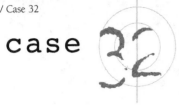

Kallmann Syndrome

Differential

Idiopathic Hypogonadotropic Hypogonadism

Erectile Dysfunction

FSH or LH Deficiency

Discussion

Kallmann syndrome is an **X-linked** disorder characterized by deficiency of GnRH with a resulting decrease in FSH and LH levels, producing an isolated hypogonadotropic hypogonadism. It is typically associated with agenesis or hypoplasia of the olfactory bulbs, producing anosmia or hyposmia (lack of stimulus for GnRH production due to absent olfactory bulb catecholamine synthesis). In idiopathic hypogonadotropic hypogonadism, the sense of smell is normal. Much more common in **men.**

Treatment

Sex steroids such as testosterone for men and estrogens and progestins for women for development of secondary sexual characteristics, gonadotropins for fertility; first human chorionic gonadotropin.

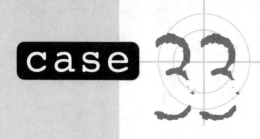
ID/CC   An 18-month-old female is taken to the emergency
        room because of **persistent vomiting** (20 times in
        24 hours) that has been unresponsive to intramuscu-
        lar antiemetics.

HPI   While on a family vacation in Mexico, she was given
        vanilla ice cream that was sold by a street vendor
        (dairy and meat products may harbor staphylococcal
        enterotoxins that produce food poisoning).

PE   VS: tachycardia; mild fever; hypotension. PE: low uri-
        nary volume; **eyes sunken; poor skin turgor** with
        dryness of skin and mucous membranes; **lethargy and
        proximal muscle weakness** (due to hypokalemia).

Labs   CBC: increased hematocrit (due to hemoconcentration);
        increased BUN. Lytes: **hypokalemia;** hypochloremia.
        UA: proteinuria; **high specific gravity.** ABGs: **meta-
        bolic alkalosis.** ECG: ST-segment and T-wave depres-
        sion; U waves (hypokalemia).

ENDOCRINOLOGY

case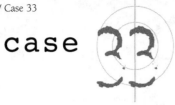

Metabolic Alkalosis

Differential

Bartter Syndrome
Pyloric Stenosis
Primary Aldosteronism
Milk-Alkali Syndrome

Discussion

Metabolic alkalosis is most commonly due to protracted vomiting but may also be caused by diuretics, volume contraction, Cushing syndrome, and congenital adrenal enzyme defects.

Breakout Point

Causes of Metabolic Alkalosis:
"CLEVER PD"   Contraction   Licorice   Endocrine (Conn, Cushing, Bartter syndromes)   Vomiting   Refeeding Alkalosis   Posthypercapnia   Diuretics

Treatment

Fluid and electrolyte replacement featuring chloride solutions (ammonium chloride or hydrochloric acid) for rapid correction from gastric chloride loss. For chloride-resistant metabolic alkalosis, carbonic anhydrase inhibitors such as acetazolamide are indicated.

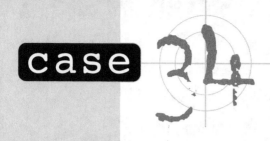

case 34

ID/CC A 72-year-old female who is a known non–insulin-dependent **diabetic** (NIDDM **type II,** maturity onset) and who has been receiving an oral hypoglycemic agent is brought to the emergency room in a **stuporous state.**

HPI For approximately 2 weeks she had been treated for a **URI** with oral antibiotics and bronchodilators.

PE VS: **tachycardia;** hypotension. PE: severe **dehydration** with dry oral mucosa and low urinary volume; patient **semiconscious** and **confused;** pupils react bilaterally and normally to light; evidence of proliferative diabetic retinopathy on funduscopic exam; no focal neurologic deficit found.

Labs CBC: mild leukocytosis (12,600). **Markedly increased blood glucose** (900 mg/dL); **increased serum and urinary osmolality** (>350 mOsm/kg). Lytes: hypernatremia; mild hypokalemia. **Normal anion gap.** ABGs: normal serum bicarbonate (no acidosis). Elevated BUN and serum creatinine (suggestive of prerenal azotemia). UA: **glycosuria with no ketonuria.**

case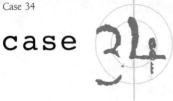

Nonketotic Hyperosmolar Coma

Differential

Diabetic Ketoacidosis

Dementia

Delirium

Discussion

Hyperosmolar, hyperglycemic nonketotic coma occurs mainly in older NIDDM patients and is usually associated with an episode of physical or mental stress (check for silent MI); it is not associated with ketosis or ketoacidosis. Coma is present in <10% of cases. Volume depletion is severe (average fluid deficit 25% of total body water), and the mortality rate is high.

Treatment

Aggressive fluid replacement, insulin infusion, potassium, and phosphate supplementation as needed.

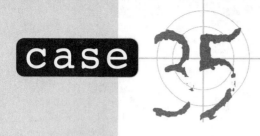
ID/CC A 47-year-old white male is admitted to the orthopedic department because he sustained a **femoral neck fracture when he fell from a small stool;** the type and magnitude of the fracture are not compatible with the patient's age and impact.

HPI The patient recently emigrated from Somalia and states that he has been suffering from increasing **leg weakness** and persistent **lower back pain.**

PE VS: normal. PE: complete right femoral neck fracture; on palpation, **tenderness of lumbar vertebrae** and pelvic rim.

Labs Mild anemia (Hb 10 g/dL). Lytes: normal. **Increased alkaline phosphatase; decreased levels of 25-OH-D$_3$; hypocalcemia; hypophosphatemia;** increased PTH.

Imaging XR:hip: surgical neck femoral fracture. XR: lumbar spine: **collapse of lumbar vertebrae; generalized osteopenia; pseudofractures** (appearance of nondisplaced fractures representing local bone resorption).

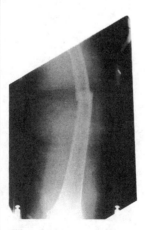

Figure 35-1. Femoral shaft fracture.

Micro Pathology Excess osteoid but poor mineralization.

ENDOCRINOLOGY

69

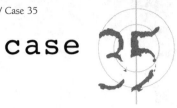

case

Osteomalacia

Differential

Osteoporosis
Secondary Hyperparathyroidism
Aneurysmal Bone Disease
Multiple Myeloma

Discussion

Renal osteodystrophy is caused by a diet poor in vitamin D and calcium, **lack of sunlight exposure, intestinal malabsorption, renal insufficiency,** or target organ resistance may lead to osteomalacia in the adult (or rickets in children), with defective calcification (incomplete mineralization) of osteoid.

Treatment

Vitamin D, calcium (and sometimes phosphate) supplements; surgical treatment of fracture, physiotherapy.

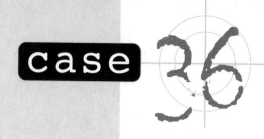
ID/CC A 41-year-old obese female comes to the ER with **severe epigastric pain radiating to the back** accompanied by nausea and vomiting; she had been advised to undergo removal of symptomatic **small gallbladder stones.**

HPI She was admitted to the surgical floor and treated for pancreatitis. On the third day, she developed **numbness of the fingers and around the mouth and tongue as well as painful leg cramps** (HYPOCALCEMIC TETANY).

PE VS: hypotension; tachycardia; fever. PE: dehydrated and in acute distress; bilateral basal hypoventilation; abdomen tender in epi-mesogastrium; facial spasm on tapping over cheek (CHVOSTEK'S SIGN); carpal spasm seen with arterial occlusion by blood pressure cuff (TROUSSEAU'S SIGN).

Labs CBC: marked leukocytosis (17,000) with neutrophilia. **Amylase and lipase markedly elevated** (due to acute pancreatitis). ECG: **Q-T prolongation.** Markedly **reduced serum calcium;** normal serum albumin.

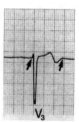

Figure 36-1. A long QT interval, comprising the duration of ventricular depolarization and repolarization, is measured from the beginning of the QRS complex to the end of the T-wave (*arrows*).

Imaging KUB: increase in gastrocolic space; **sentinel loop.** CXR: small left pleural effusion.

Gross Pathology Hemorrhagic pancreatitis with edema and areas of gray-white necrosis; intraperitoneal free hemorrhagic fluid; chalky-white fat necrosis (**saponification of calcium with lipids**).

case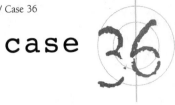

Pancreatic Hypocalcemia

Differential

Acute Pancreatitis
Acute Renal Failure
Hyperparathyroidism
Hyperphosphatemia
Hypomagnesemia

Discussion

The levels of cholesterol/triglycerides and calcium need to be determined with respect to the etiology of pancreatitis (hypercalcemia or hyperlipidemia) or complications of pancreatitis whereby there is **an obstruction or hyperdistension to the pancreatic duct. Hypocalcemia arises from fats being saponified** in the **retroperitoneum.**

Treatment

Treat pancreatitis with analgesics. IV calcium gluconate.

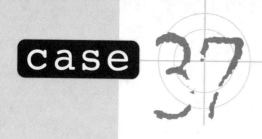

case 37

ID/CC A 42-year-old male visits his internist for an evaluation of sudden (PAROXYSMAL) **attacks of headache, perspiration (DIAPHORESIS), and anxiety;** attacks are precipitated by exercise, emotional stress, postural changes, and, at times, urination.

HPI **Very high blood pressure** has been recorded at the time of previous paroxysms. The patient has a good appetite but looks cachectic; blood pressure recorded between paroxysms is normal. The patient has no history suggestive of renal disease.

PE VS: extreme **hypertension** (BP 180/120). PE: hypertensive retinopathy changes on funduscopic exam.

Labs **Elevated blood sugar.** Lytes: normal. **Increased** 24-hour urinary free **catecholamines** and **vanillylmandelic acid (VMA)** levels.

Imaging CT/MR: 3-cm left **adrenal mass;** very high signal on T2-weighted MR.

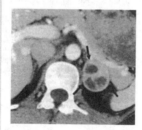

Figure 37-1. 3-cm mass in the left adrenal gland that contains focal areas of necrosis (*arrows*).

Gross Pathology Encapsulated, **dusky-colored,** round tumor mass with compressed adrenal gland remnants at periphery and foci of necrosis and hemorrhage.

Micro Pathology Nests of pleomorphic large cells with basophilic cytoplasm and **chrome-staining granules** in vascular stroma; argentaffin stains positive; membrane-bound secretory granules on electron microscopy.

ENDOCRINOLOGY

73

case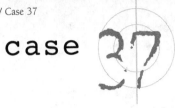

Pheochromocytoma

Differential

Adrenal Adenoma

Adrenal Carcinoma

Hyperthyroidism

Anxiety Disorders

Discussion

Pheochromocytoma is the most common **tumor of the adrenal medulla** in adults; its symptoms are produced by **increased production of catecholamines**. These tumors **secrete epinephrine >>> norepinephrine** (except in familial pheochromocytoma; Normal adrenal medulla is >80% norepinephrine), but rarely dopamine. Of these large tumors (often >3 cm), 10% are extra-adrenal, 10% bilateral, 10% malignant, and 10% familial; 10% occur in children, and 10% calcify. May be associated with multiple endocrine neoplasias (MEN) IIA or IIB syndromes.

Treatment

Treat hypertensive crises with pharmacologic alpha and beta blockade (pretreat with low doses of alpha blockers [Phenoxybenzamine hydrochloride is longer acting, Doxazosin mesylate inhibits post synaptic receptors] as monotherapy prior to beta blockers); resection of tumor.

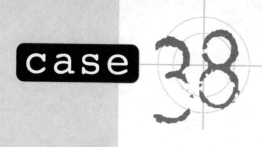

case 38

ID/CC
A **6-year-old** black female is brought to her pediatrician because of **breast enlargement.**

HPI
Her mother also reports **cyclical vaginal bleeding** and the appearance of **pubic and axillary hair** since the age of 4; an older cousin developed similar signs and symptoms.

PE
Fully developed breasts; axillary and pubic hair present; clitoral enlargement; normal mental development; height and weight greater than average for her age; no focal neurologic signs.

Labs
Increased plasma FSH, LH, and estradiol; pubertal pattern of increased gonadotropins after infusion of GnRH.

Imaging
XR: **advanced bone age.** US: ovary enlarged to pubertal size with cyst formation. CT/MR: no pituitary lesion.

Gross Pathology
Ovarian cyst formation (luteal); in idiopathic variety, no structural abnormality found.

ENDOCRINOLOGY

case 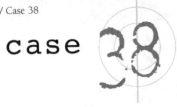 38

Precocious Puberty

Differential 3-β Hydroxysteroid Dehydrogenase Deficiency
Congenital Adrenal Hyperplasia
Granulosa Cell Tumor
Virilizing Adrenal Tumor
McCune-Albright Syndrome
Leydig Cell Tumor

Discussion The most common cause of central precocious puberty is idiopathic or constitutional; less common causes include hypothalamic-pituitary tumors (pinealomas, hamartomas, gliomas) or lesions causing gonadotropin-dependent precocious puberty. Precocious pseudopuberty results from a gonadotropin independent production of sex steroids.

TABLE 38-1 Precocious or Inappropriate Sexual Development

True or central precocious puberty (central gonadotropin secretion)	Congenital adrenal hyperplasia
Idiopathic	Adrenal tumors
Central nervous system tumors: hamartomas, gliomas (with neurofibromatosis), and others	Testicular androgen secretion Tumors Familial Leydig cell hyperplasia
Other central nervous system disorders: trauma, postinfectious, hydrocephalus, radiation, surgery	Gonadotropin-secreting tumors McCune-Albright syndrome
Severe primary hypothyroidism	**Heterosexual development**
Precocious puberty independent of pituitary gonadotropins	Virilization in girls Congenital adrenal hyperplasia
Girls	Adrenal tumors
Exogenous estrogen exposure	Ovarian tumors
Estrogen-secreting tumors (adrenals or ovaries)	Feminization in boys Adrenal tumor
Ovarian cysts	Testicular tumor
McCune-Albright syndrome	Increased peripheral conversion of androgens to estrogens
Boys	**Variations of normal puberty**
Exogenous androgen exposure	Premature thelarche
Adrenal androgen secretion	Premature adrenarche
	Pubertal gynecomastia

Treatment GnRH agonists (Leuprolide, Nafarelin); psychosocial support; continuous search for possible cause.

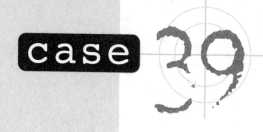
ID/CC A 5-year-old female is brought to the pediatrician because of intermittent **numbness and leg cramps**.

HPI Her parents are concerned about the fact that their child is **shorter** than her classmates.

PE **Full, round face;** short neck; flat nasal bridge; right convergence squint and left **cataract; delayed dentition;** positive Chvostek's and Trousseau's signs.

Labs CBC: normal. Lytes: **hypocalcemia** (>8.8 mg/dL); **hyperphosphatemia** (>5 mg/dL). **Increased** plasma PTH; **no increase** in renal **cAMP** and phosphate clearance **with PTH infusion.**

Imaging XR: **fourth and fifth metacarpals** are **short; premature physeal closure;** thickening of cortices with demineralization.

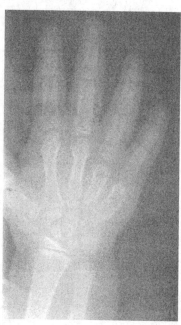

Figure 39-1. Shortened fourth and fifth metacarpals.

ENDOCRINOLOGY

77

case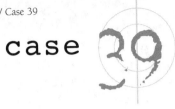

Pseudohypoparathyroidism

Differential
Secondary Hyperparathyroidism
Vitamin D Deficiency
Autoimmune Polyglandular Syndrome

Discussion
Pseudohypoparathyroidism is a heterogeneous group of hereditary disorders in which there is **resistance to PTH action on the renal tubule** and bone with resulting hypocalcemia. At least two types exist according to the response of cAMP to PTH. In type I (as in this case), patients fail to exhibit a phosphaturic response or increased cAMP after administration of PTH. Type II is associated with Albright's hereditary osteodystrophy.

Treatment
Calcitriol and calcium supplementation to correct calcium deficiency.

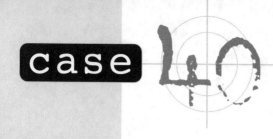

case 40

ID/CC A 72-year-old male smoker presents with headache, weakness, **fatigue**, and **decreased urinary output** (OLIGURIA).

HPI He was recently diagnosed with **oat cell carcinoma of the lung**.

PE Cardiac sounds normal; no murmurs; no arrhythmias; no pitting edema; no hepatomegaly; no jugular plethora (no evidence of cardiac disease); no asterixis, jaundice, spider nevi, or parotid enlargement (no evidence of hepatic disease).

Labs **Decreased serum sodium** (HYPONATREMIA); **decreased serum osmolality** (<280 mOsm/kg); normal or low BUN and serum creatinine; no proteinuria (no renal disease); adrenal and thyroid function tests normal. UA: **urine osmolality markedly increased** (versus psychogenic polydipsia where osmolality is decreased); hypernatriuria (urinary Na >20 mEq/L). **Diminished blood uric acid level** (HYPOURICEMIA).

ENDOCRINOLOGY

79

case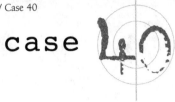

SIADH—Syndrome of Inappropriate Antidiuretic Hormone Secretion

Differential
Hyponatremia
Adrenal Insufficiency
Hypothyroidism
Renal Failure

Discussion
Syndrome of inappropriate (increased) secretion of **antidiuretic hormone** (SIADH) occurs with either increased hypothalamic secretion (e.g., CNS disease, postoperative states) or ectopic secretion (e.g., tumors such as oat cell carcinoma of the lung). There may also be increased sensitivity to the effect of ADH (with chlorpropamide, fluoxetine, and carbamazepine).

Breakout Point

Causes of SIADH:
Surgery   **I**ntracranial: infection, head injury, CVA   **A**lveolar: Cancer   **D**rugs: opiates, antiepileptics, cytotoxics, antipsychotics   **H**ormonal: hypothyroid, low corticosteroid level

Treatment
Water restriction, and if refractory, tetracycline such as demeclocycline. Arginine vasopressin receptor 2 antagonists (Conivaptan).

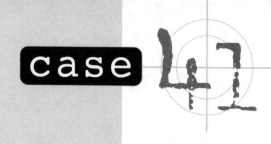

case 47

ID/CC A **50-year-old white male** presents with **decreased libido, progressive impotence, fatigue,** and **muscle weakness** (loss of strength).

HPI He underwent a **transsphenoidal hypophysectomy** for a **large pituitary tumor** 2 months ago. He is currently on hormone replacement therapy with thyroxine and corticosteroids.

PE VS: normal. PE: bilateral **breast enlargement** (GYNECOMASTIA), **bilateral testicular atrophy,** and **loss of facial and pubic hair.**

Labs **Decreased serum testosterone level; decreased serum LH and FSH.**

case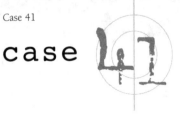

Testosterone Deficiency

Differential

Hypogonadism (see discussion)

3-ß-Hydroxysteroid Dehydrogenase Deficiency

Discussion

Hypogonadism or **testosterone deficiency** is either congenital or acquired. Causes are categorized as either **primary** (hypergonadotropic, high FSH/LH levels) or **secondary** (hypogonadotropic, low FSH/LH levels). The most common congenital cause of primary hypogonadism is Klinefelter syndrome. Acquired causes include trauma, surgery, testicular torsion, irradiation, chemotherapy, alcoholism, and aging. Secondary hypogonadism is associated with disorders such as Kallmann and Prader–Willi syndromes or with pituitary tumors or trauma. Side effects of testosterone include **itching** and **local irritation** (when given topically) and **liver dysfunction** and a **decrease in HDL** (when given orally). Testosterone is contraindicated in men with prostatic carcinoma.

Treatment

Testosterone replacement via either a transdermal testosterone or IM injections; long-term use of testosterone produces subjective improvement in mood, energy, libido, muscle mass and strength, and sexual function.

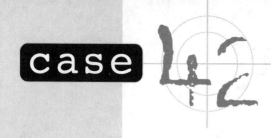

case 42

ID/CC   A 44-year-old Hispanic female is brought by ambulance to the emergency room from her workplace because of **confusion, agitation,** diarrhea, and **vomiting.**

HPI   She gives a history of **recent weight loss** (7 kg) and a **recent severe URI.**

PE   VS: **fever** (39.3°C); **tachycardia** with irregular pulse; hypotension (BP 100/50); **hypermetabolic.** PE: irritability; **delirium;** exophthalmos; diffuse increase in size of thyroid gland (GOITER); lungs clear; abdomen soft and nontender; no masses; no peritoneal irritation; deep tendon reflexes brisk; no neck stiffness or focal neurologic signs.

Labs   CBC/Lytes: normal. LP: CSF values normal. ECG: atrial fibrillation. **Elevated T_4, free T_4, and T_3; low TSH.**

case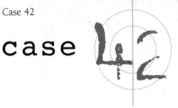

Thyroid Storm

Differential
Hyperthyroidism
Graves Disease
Pheochromocytoma
Supraventricular Tachycardia

Discussion
Thyroid storm, a medical emergency, is usually precipitated by surgical or medical stress (e.g., infection) placed on untreated or undertreated hyperthyroid patients with excess circulating thyroid hormone (**thyrotoxicosis**). Diffuse toxic goiter (Graves disease) is an autoimmune condition. Prevention of postoperative crises is effected through use of iodine and antithyroid drugs.

Breakout Point

> **"Storm HITS":**
>
> Thyroid **storm** due to:
> **H**yperthyroidism
> **I**nfection or **I**llness at childbirth
> **T**rauma
> **S**urgery

Treatment
Treatment involves inhibition of thyroid hormone synthesis (propylthiouracil or methimazole); inhibition of stored thyroid hormone release (iodide and corticosteroids); suppression of the peripheral effects of thyroid hormone with beta-blockers (propranolol); digitalization of patients with CHF and atrial fibrillation; acetaminophen for fever; and treatment of precipitating factors (e.g., antibiotics for infections).

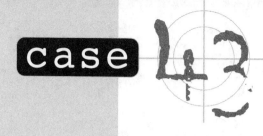

case 42

ID/CC A 25-year-old white **female of Swedish nationality** is brought to the ER because of strange, dreamlike **hallucinations and blurred vision** that she experienced one day **after spending all morning in the sun** painting her house (exposure to sun may precipitate attacks).

HPI The patient had undergone two **previous laparotomies** for apparent acute abdomen, but **no pathology was found.** She has had several episodes of **recurrent abdominal pain.**

PE VS: no fever but evidence of slight tachycardia. PE: pupils are of unequal size (ANISOCORIA); generalized weakness and hypoactive deep-tendon reflexes; disorientation; **foot drop; urine very dark** and foulsmelling. No photosensitive skin lesions. Some **peripheral neuropathy** is present.

Labs UA: **increased urine porphobilinogen** and **gammaaminolevulinic acid.** Lytes: hyponatremia.

Gross Pathology Liver infiltrated with porphobilinogen; central and peripheral nervous system myelin sheath degeneration.

Micro Pathology Axonal degeneration and myelin sheath degradation.

case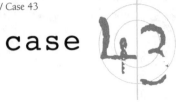

Acute Intermittent Porphyria

Differential | Diverticulitis
Irritable Bowel Syndrome
Lead Neuropathy
Fibromyalgia

Discussion | Acute intermittent porphyria is an **autosomal-dominant deficiency** in an enzyme of porphyrin metabolism (**porphobilinogen deaminase**) that leads to systemic symptoms, acute abdominal pain, neuropsychiatric signs and symptoms, and CNS and peripheral neuropathy. Acute intermittent porphyria is differentiated from other porphyrias by its **lack of photosensitive skin lesions.** Sun exposure and drugs (e.g., sulfa, barbiturates) may precipitate attacks, but in general patients are not photosensitive.

TABLE 43-1 CLINICAL FEATURES OF PORPHYRIA

Type of porphyria	Usual inheritance	Neurologic dysfunction	Photocutaneous lesion	Structural liver disease	Hepatocellular carcinoma
Acute intermittent porphyria	AD	+	−	−	+
Variegate porphyria	AD	+	+	−	+
Hereditary coproporphyria	AD	+	+	−	−
ALA dehydrase deficiency	AR	+	−	−	−
Porphyria cutanea tarda	AD (familial type)	−	+	+	+
Hepatoerythropoietic porphyria	AR	−	+	±	−
Congenital erythropoietic porphyria	AR	−	+	−	−
Protoporphyria	AD	−	+	+	−

AD, autosomal dominant; AR, autosomal recessive.

Treatment | Pharmacotherapy involves inhibiting heme synthesis with hemin; remove offending medications; control of pain, nausea, and vomiting.

case

ID/CC A 56-year-old male accountant visits his internist because of episodic **watery diarrhea** accompanied by wheezing, palpitations, and facial flushing.

HPI When working or exercising in the sun, he develops a rash on exposed areas (PHOTODERMATITIS).

PE VS: normal. PE: in no acute distress; **hot red flushing of face;** no neck masses or increased JVP; **systolic ejection murmur grade I/IV at pulmonary area,** increasing with inspiration (pulmonary stenosis); wheezing heard; abdomen soft and nontender; mild **hepatomegaly.**

Labs CBC/Lytes: normal. Glucose, BUN, creatinine, and LFTs normal; no ova or parasites in stool. UA: **increased 5-hydroxyindoleacetic acid (5-HIAA) in urine.**

Imaging KUB: ladder-step air-fluid levels. UGI: small bowel loops kinked, causing obstruction.

Micro Pathology Argentophilic cells (KULCHITSKY CELLS) in the intestinal crypts of Lieberkühn invading into mesentery; marked fibrotic reaction. Highly vascularized.

case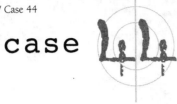

Carcinoid Syndrome

Differential

Irritable Bowel Syndrome
Anaphylaxis
Ogilvie Syndrome
Pellegra

Discussion

Carcinoid tumors arise from the gastrointestinal tract or bronchi. These tumors secrete **serotonin** (5-HYDROXYTRYPTAMINE), producing the typical clinical syndrome. There may be stenosis of the pulmonic and tricuspid valve and **right-sided heart failure.**

Breakout Point

> **CARCINOID 1/3 RULE:**
>
> **1/3** are multiple tumors
> **1/3** of those in the GI tract are in the small bowel
> **1/3** metastasize
> **1/3** have a second malignancy

Treatment

Surgical resection, when possible, is curative. Octreotide, cyproheptadine (SOMATOSTATIN ANALOG).

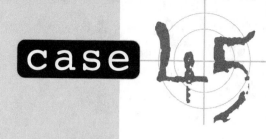

case 45

ID/CC A 3-week-old male is seen by a neonatologist because of **severe jaundice** that appeared at birth and has been worsening ever since.

HPI He is the first-born child of a healthy **Jewish** couple. His mother had an uneventful pregnancy and delivery.

PE Average weight and height for age; in no acute distress; **marked jaundice** (jaundice appears at levels of bilirubin around 2.5 to 3.0 mg/dL); slight hepatomegaly.

Labs **Markedly increased serum unconjugated bilirubin** (20 mg/dL); **very low fecal urobilinogen;** decreased uridyl glucuronyl transferase activity on liver biopsy.

case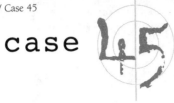

Crigler–Najjar Syndrome

Differential | Gilbert Syndrome
Neonatal Jaundice
Breast Milk Jaundice
Hemolytic Disorders

Discussion | Crigler–Najjar syndrome is an inherited disorder of bilirubin metabolism that is characterized by a **deficiency** of the enzyme **glucuronyl transferase** and hence by an inability to conjugate bilirubin, with accumulation of indirect bilirubin and risk of kernicterus with brain damage (at bilirubin concentrations of >20 mg/dL). There are two types: type I, which is more severe and is autosomal recessive, and type II (Arias syndrome), which is autosomal dominant with low levels of UGT-1 enzyme that can be induced with phenobarbital.

■ TABLE 45-1 CLASSIFICATION OF CONJUGATED HYPERBILIRUBINEMIAS

Impaired canalicular excretion
    Hepatocellular injury (e.g., viral hepatitis, alcoholic hepatitis, cirrhosis)
    Intrahepatic cholestasis (e.g., intrahepatic cholestasis of pregnancy, total parenteral nutrition-induced jaundice)
    Familial disorders of conjugated bilirubin transport (Dubin-Johnson and Rotor syndromes)

Disorders of the intrahepatic bile ducts
    Primary biliary cirrhosis
    Primary sclerosing cholangitis
    Liver allograft rejection
    Graft versus host disease
    Neoplasms

Disorders of the extrahepatic ducts
    Choledocholithiasis
    Neoplasms
    Primary sclerosing cholangitis
    Biliary strictures

Treatment | Plasma exchange transfusion; long-term phototherapy; **liver transplantation,** barbiturates to attenuate neurological effects (Phenobarbital).

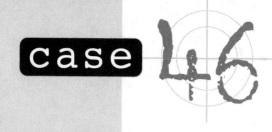

case 46

ID/CC	A 21-year-old female college student visits her gastroenterologist for an evaluation of fatigability and intermittent **right upper quadrant and epigastric pain.**
HPI	She asked her family doctor to refer her to a gastroenterologist because she was concerned about her pain despite her doctor's reassurance that it was "nothing important."
PE	VS: normal. PE: mild **jaundice** in conjunctiva and underneath tongue; well hydrated and in no acute distress; no hepatosplenomegaly on abdominal exam; no signs of hepatic failure.
Labs	**Increased direct bilirubin** (vs. Gilbert syndrome, in which hyperbilirubinemia is indirect) **and indirect bilirubin; liver enzymes mildly elevated.** UA: bilirubin and urobilinogen (vs. Gilbert syndrome); **ratio of coproporphyrin I and coproporphyrin III in urine 5:1** (normal <1).
Imaging	US: no gallstones; liver normal. Nuc: prolonged visualization of liver without visualization of gallbladder is characteristic on HIDA.
Gross Pathology	**Liver** normal size and areas of **dark green pigmentation;** absence of gallbladder inflammation or stones.

case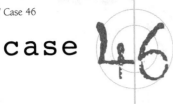

Dubin–Johnson Syndrome

Differential   Rotor Syndrome

Conjugated Hyperbilirubinemia

Discussion   Dubin–Johnson syndrome is a benign **autosomal-recessive** disorder (vs. Gilbert syndrome) of **defective canalicular bilirubin excretion** characterized by episodes of intermittent jaundice.

Treatment   Supportive, this is a benign disorder.

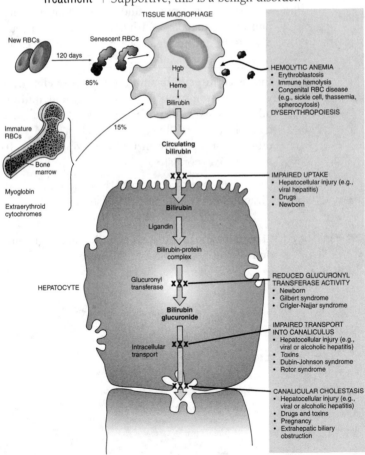

Figure 46-1. Mechanisms of jaundice.

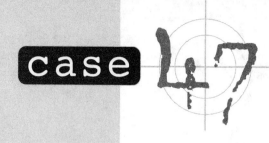

case 47

ID/CC A 17-year-old white male with a URI visits his family doctor because he is concerned about **yellowness in his eyes** (JAUNDICE), which he has noticed **whenever he is fatigued** or is suffering from a minor infection.

HPI He has no history of dark-colored urine, clay-colored stools, abdominal pain, blood transfusions, or drug use. He is immunized against hepatitis B and does not drink alcohol.

PE **Normal except for mild scleral icterus**; no hepatosplenomegaly; no signs of chronic liver failure.

Labs CBC/PBS: **normal.** Reticulocyte count **normal**; LDH normal; moderately **increased serum bilirubin, predominantly unconjugated**; normal serum transaminases and alkaline phosphatase; normal serum albumin; **serum bilirubin rises after 24-hour fast.**

case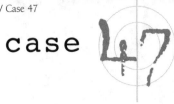

Gilbert Disease

Differential
Hemolysis

Acute Liver Disease

Crigler-Najjar Syndrome Type II

Discussion
The most common example of idiopathic (unconjugated) hyperbilirubinemia is Gilbert disease, which is autosomal dominant with variable penetrance. It is due to **defective bilirubin uptake by liver cells** and **low glucuronyl transferase activity.** Bilirubin levels seldom exceed 5 mg/dL, mainly unconjugated, and may vary inversely with caloric intake.

Treatment
Reassurance that there is no increased morbidity; no medical treatment necessary. Avoid fasting and dehydration.

■ **TABLE 47-1 CLASSIFICATION OF UNCONJUGATED HYPERBILIRUBINEMIAS**

Increased bilirubin production
 Hemolysis
 Ineffective erythropoiesis

Impaired bilirubin uptake
 Gilbert syndrome
 Drugs (e.g., rifampin, radiographic contrast agents, flavispidic acid)
 Congestive heart failure
 Surgical or spontaneous portosystemic shunts
 Neonatal jaundice

Impaired bilirubin conjugation
 Gilbert syndrome
 Crigler-Najjar syndrome
 Neonatal jaundice

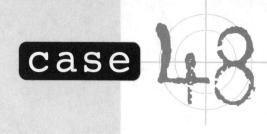

case 48

ID/CC	A 19-year-old female is brought to her family doctor by her parents, who have noticed that she has started **behaving oddly**; 2 days ago they noticed that her **eyes were yellow**.
HPI	She also complains of **tremor of her hands at rest** and some **rigidity** when trying to grasp objects (basal ganglia affectation). The **parents** of the patient are **first cousins**.
PE	Patient shows flapping tremor (ASTERIXIS) of hands; slit-lamp examination reveals **copper deposits in Descemet's membrane** of the cornea (KAYSER–FLEISCHER RINGS).
Labs	CBC: hemolytic anemia (due to oxidative RBC damage by copper). **AST and ALT elevated** as well as alkaline phosphatase and bilirubin, both direct and indirect; **decrease in serum ceruloplasmin** (copper-transporting protein); **increased urinary copper** (HYPERCUPRIURIA).
Imaging	MR: low signal intensity on T1-weighting in white matter, pons, and deep cerebellar areas
Gross Pathology	Copper accumulation in liver, brain, and cornea.
Micro Pathology	Liver biopsy shows acute inflammation, increased copper levels, and periportal fibrosis (macronodular cirrhosis); **intracytoplasmic hyaline bodies** (MALLORY BODIES) seen; **degeneration of basal ganglia with cavitation especially of putamen; hyperplasia with glial proliferation of the lenticular nuclie.**

case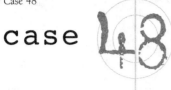

Wilson Disease

Differential | Anemia
Hemochromatosis
Viral Hepatitis
Schizophrenia

Discussion | Wilson disease (hepatolenticular degeneration) is an **autosomal-recessive** inherited disorder of copper metabolism resulting in a **neurodegenerative disease**. It is characterized by **increased absorption of copper from the intestine and diminished excretion in the bile** with resultant copper deposition, primarily in the brain and liver.

Treatment | **Penicillamine** (copper chelating drug), pyridoxine. Consider liver transplantation for fulminant hepatic failure and end-stage cirrhosis.

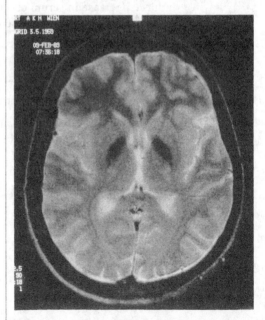

Figure 48-1. Bilateral hyperintense thalamic lesions are hypointense on T1 weighted images in Wilson Disease.

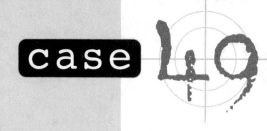

case 49

ID/CC A 27-year-old **farmer from Florida** (with abundant sun exposure) comes to see his dermatologist for an evaluation of a recent **increase in size and change in color of a skin lesion** that has been present on the dorsum of his hand (a sun-exposed area) for 6 years.

HPI The patient is **extremely light skinned**, but he has not been able to comply with his dermatologist's orders to wear long sleeves while working in the field.

PE **White hair, including eyelashes and eyebrows;** eye exam shows **nystagmus** and poor development of macula with blue iris; poor visual acuity (20/350); skin is pink-white with lack of pigmentation throughout body; numerous actinic (SOLAR) keratoses on face and scalp as well as on dorsum of hands; **ulcerated lesion with indurated edges** on dorsum of hand with hyperpigmentation.

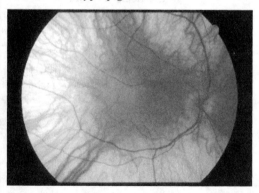

Figure 49-1. Fundoscopic exam: Note absence of pigment and prominence of choroidal vasculature.

Labs **Tyrosine** assay shows **absence** of the enzyme.

Gross Pathology Patches of scaly, irregular, hypertrophied skin in sun-exposed areas (**actinic keratosis**).

Micro Pathology Biopsy of lesion on dorsum of hand shows epidermoid (**squamous cell**) cancer with epithelial pearls.

97

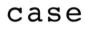

case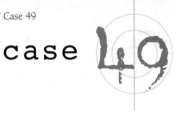

Albinism

Differential

Ichthyosis
Hermansky-Pudlak Syndrome
Phenylketonuria
Homocysteinuria
Menkes Kinky Hair Disease

Discussion

Albinism is a hereditary disorder that may be generalized or localized and is transmitted as either an autosomal-dominant or autosomal-recessive trait. The heterogeneous phenotype reflects where mutations occur along the **melanin** pathway. It is always distinguished by various degrees of **hypopigmentation** of the skin, hair, iris, and retina. The defect lies in the pigmentation, not in the number of melanocytes present in the body. The cause is an **absence of tyrosinase,** the enzyme that catalyzes the conversion of tyrosine to dihydroxyphenylalanine and melanin. There is a marked increase in the risk of skin cancer.

Treatment

Surgery and/or chemotherapy for skin cancers, avoidance of sun exposure, management of visual impairment.

case 50

ID/CC	A 37-year-old man presents with **dark, blackened spots in his sclera and ear cartilage** as well as **back pain** and restriction of motion with **pain and swelling of both knee joints.**
HPI	Directed questioning reveals that his **urine turns black** if left standing.
PE	**Increased pigmentation** in ears, conjunctiva, nasal bridge, neck, and anterior thorax (OCHRONOSIS); arthritis of spine, both knee joints, and fingers.
Labs	UA: **elevated urine homogentisic acid** (urine darkens upon standing or with addition of alkaline substances). ECG: no contraindications.
Gross Pathology	Deposition of dark pigmentation in sclera, cartilage, and synovial membranes.

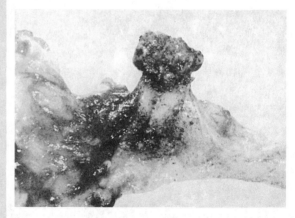

Figure 50-1. Deposition of dark pigmentation on synovial tissue.

Imaging	XR: calcification in cartilage of knee menisci and wrist; premature arthritic changes. CXR: negative for aortic or mitral valve stenosis.

case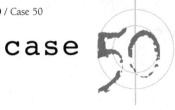

Alkaptonuria

Differential

Acute Porphyria

Osteoarthritis

Argyria

Arsenical Keratosis

Discussion

Also called **ochronosis,** alkaptonuria is an autosomal-recessive disorder of tyrosine metabolism characterized by the **absence of homogentisate oxidase** due to a defective gene on chromosome 3 with accumulation of homogentisic acid in cartilage, giving a dark blue discoloration to the tissues and leading to degenerative joint disease.

Treatment

Symptomatic treatment of arthritis. Supplemental vitamin C.

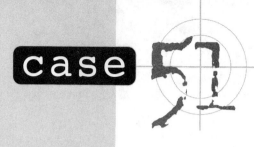

ID/CC
An **11-year-old white** female is brought to the ER by her parents because of fever, **difficulty breathing, and a productive cough with greenish sputum.**

HPI
Her parents are of northern European descent. She has a history of **recurrent** lower respiratory tract infections **and foul-smelling diarrhea** since infancy.

PE
VS: tachycardia; tachypnea (RR 45). PE: mild cyanosis; malnourishment; clubbing of fingernails; **nasal polyps;** hyperresonance to lung percussion with **barrel-shaped chest;** scattered rales; hepatomegaly.

Labs
High sodium and chloride concentrations in **sweat test;** *Pseudomonas aeruginosa, Haemophilus influenzae,* and *Staphylococcus aureus* in sputum culture. PFTs: increased RV/TLC ratio. Increased **fecal fat.** ABGs: hypoxemia; hypercapnia.

Imaging
CXR: few dilated bronchi (BRONCHIECTASIS) filled with mucus; peribronchial thickening; emphysema; XR: paranasal sinuses: opacification of sinuses.

Gross Pathology
Atrophic pancreas with almost complete disruption of acini and replacement of exocrine pancreas with fibrous tissue and fat; mucous plugging of canaliculi.

Micro Pathology
Inflammatory changes.

case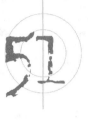

Cystic Fibrosis

Differential

Failure to Thrive

Asthma

Aspergillosis

Kartagener Syndrome

Celiac Disease

Discussion

Cystic fibrosis (CF) is the most common lethal inherited disease in whites. Cystic fibrosis is an **autosomal-recessive** disease due to a mutation (508delF is the most common mutation), in the long arm of **chromosome 7** (band q31) in the cystic fibrosis transmembrane conductance regulator (**CFTR**) gene encoding a **cyclic AMP-regulated chloride channel.** If CFTR function is deficient, **chloride** and water transport is slowed and secretions are inspissated. End stage, progressive lung disease is the principle cause of death.

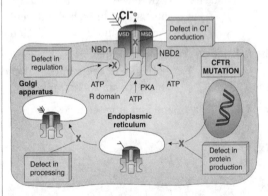

Figure 51-1. Cellular sites of the disruptions in the synthesis and function of CFTR in CF.

Treatment

Antibiotics for pneumonia; bronchodilation, breathing exercises, and chest physiotherapy to clear secretions; recombinant DNase and mucolytics; pancreatic enzyme replacement (Pancrelipase); adequate nutritional support including fat soluble vitamins (A, D, E, K); liver, lung, pancreas transplantation.

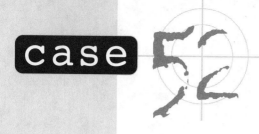
ID/CC A 15-year-old white female is brought to the emergency room from school following the sudden development of **severe, intermittent right-flank pain** together with nausea, vomiting, and **blood in her urine** (typical of renoureteral stone).

HPI Her medical and family history is unremarkable.

PE VS: tachycardia; normal BP; slight fever. PE: short stature (due to lysine deficiency); in acute distress; **constantly switches positions in bed** (due to renal colic); abdominal tenderness; no peritoneal irritation; costovertebral angle tenderness.

Labs **Increased urinary excretion of cysteine and dibasic amino acids (ornithine, arginine, and lysine)** on urine amino acid chromatography (due to intestinal and renal **defect in reabsorption**).

Imaging KUB/IVP/CT urography: radiopaque stone in area of right kidney.

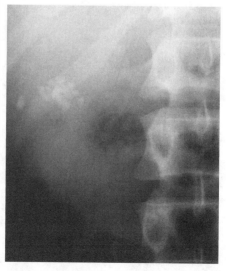

Figure 52-1. Radiopaque cluster of stones in kidney

103

case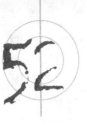

Cystinuria

Differential

Wilson Disease
Hypercalcemia
Hyperuricemia
Hartnup Disease

Discussion

Cystinuria is an **autosomal-recessive** disorder of cystine dibasic amino acid metabolism (due to a mutation in *SLC3A1* the gene encoding the renal basic amino acid transporter, thus impairing renal tubular reabsorption); it leads to increased cysteine urinary excretion and **kidney stone formation.**

Treatment

Low-methionine diet; low sodium diet (decreasing cystine excretion), increase fluid intake; alkalinize urine; penicillamine, alpha-mercaptopropionylglycine, captopril, or other cystine chelating agent. Large calculi require surgery.

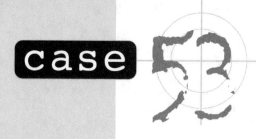

case 53

ID/CC A 9-year-old boy is brought to the emergency room with pain, inability to move his left shoulder, and flattening of the normal rounded shoulder contour (SHOULDER DISLOCATION) that occurred when he tried to hit a ball with his bat at a local baseball field.

HPI He has **dislocated his left shoulder nine times before and his right shoulder three times before.** He also has a history of **easy bruising.**

PE **Hyperelastic skin;** "**cigarette paper**" scars in areas of trauma; **hyperextensibility of joints;** left shoulder dislocated; multiple bruises over skin.

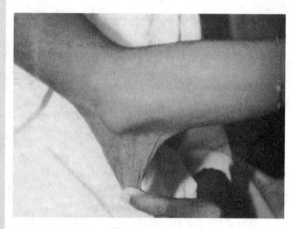

Figure 53-1. Hyperextensibile skin.

Labs Clotting profile normal.

Imaging XR: left shoulder dislocated.

Micro Pathology Collagen fibrils of dermis of skin larger than normal and irregular in outline on electron microscopy.

case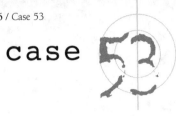

Ehlers–Danlos Syndrome

Differential	Williams Syndrome
	Turner Syndrome
	Cutis Laxis
	Pseudoxanthoma Elasticum
Discussion	Ehlers–Danlos syndrome is a group of diseases due to a genetic **defect in collagen chain synthesis or assembly** and exhibits attenuated tensile strength of joints, skin, and other connective tissues. Ten subtypes are known; **"classic" type I** is the most common type following an autosomal-dominant mode of inheritance with skin hyperextensibility, joint hypermobility causing mitral valve prolapse, and premature rupture of fetal membranes. **"Vascular" type IV** is an autosomal-recessive disease characterized by abnormal type III collagen, resulting is spontaneous, life-threatening arterial and bowel ruptures, and life expectancy with this form is reduced.
Treatment	Supportive. Improvement of wound healing with vitamin C has been indicated.

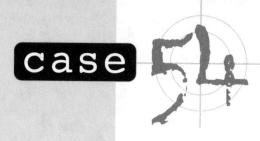

ID/CC A 17-year-old **male** presents with episodes of **painful, burning paresthesias along his palms and soles** along with markedly **diminished vision** in his right eye.

HPI His maternal **uncle died of chronic renal failure** at the age of 40.

PE Clusters of **purplish-red, hyperkeratotic lesions** on skin around umbilicus, buttocks, and scrotum (ANGIOKERATOMAS); **right corneal leukomatous opacity**; neurologic exam normal except for painful paresthesias along arms and soles; pitting edema in lower extremities.

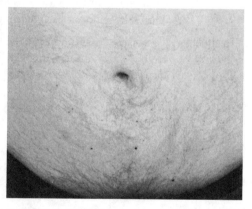

Figure 54-1. Angiokeratomas.

Labs **Elevated serum creatinine and BUN** (patients usually die of renal failure). UA: proteinuria; broad casts. PBS: leukocytes reveal deficiency of α-galactosidase; **alpha-galactosidase A** activity was 5% normal.

Micro Pathology Lipid deposition in epithelial and endothelial cells of glomeruli and tubules (FOAM CELLS) on renal biopsy; **lysosomal accumulation of glycosphingolipid (ceramide trihexoside)** in the form of "myelin bodies" on electron microscopy of skin, heart, kidneys, and CNS.

107

case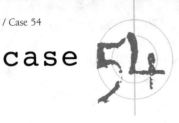

Fabry Disease

Differential

Galactokinase Deficiency

Acute Stroke

Posterior Cerebral Artery Stroke

Dissection Syndrome

Discussion

Fabry disease, a lysosomal storage disease, is a **rare X-linked recessive disorder** of glycosphingolipid metabolism (sphingolipidosis) caused by a **deficiency of alpha-galactosidase A** and by the consequent **accumulation of ceramide trihexosides** in kidney, heart, and nervous system. Glycosphingolipids are components of the plasma membrane that are internalized by endocytosis and degraded in the lysosome.

Treatment

Treat pain crises symptomatically; renal failure may require renal transplantation. In 2006, enzyme replacement therapy with Agalsidase beta was implemented.

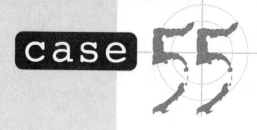

ID/CC An 8-year-old Jewish boy is referred to the pediatric clinic for evaluation of **anemia and multiple developmental anomalies.**

HPI His parents report that he **bleeds easily.**

PE Pale and **mentally retarded**; small head (MICRO-CEPHALIA); low height and weight for age; hyperpigmentation of torso and thighs with café-au-lait spots; **decrease in size of penis**; decrease in size of eyes (MICROPHTHALMIA); **absence of both thumbs.**

Labs CBC: decreased WBCs (LEUKOPENIA), platelets (THROMBOCYTOPENIA), and RBCs (ANEMIA) (PANCYTOPENIA). Increased levels of HbF; bone marrow biopsy hypocellular in myeloid, erythroid, and megakaryocyte lines; chromosome breakage studies of lymphocytes positive.

Imaging XR: **bilateral absence of radii.** IVP/CT: **hypoplastic kidneys.**

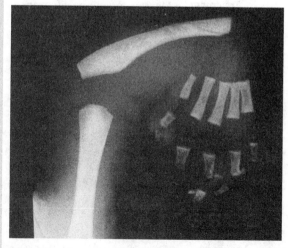

Figure 55-1. Absence of radial bones.

case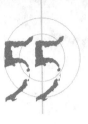

Fanconi Anemia

Differential	Shwachman-Diamond Syndrome
	Myelodysplastic Syndrome
	Pearson Syndrome
	Wermer Syndrome
	Teratogen Exposure

Discussion Fanconi anemia (FA) is a congenital, autosomal-recessive disorder of one of 11 genes (*FANCA* through *FANCJ; FANCD1* is *BRCA2*), characterized by constitutional **aplastic anemia due to defective DNA repair,** causing hypersensitivity to DNA cross-linking agents. It is associated with multiple musculoskeletal visceral anomalies and proximal renal tubular acidosis. Complications include infection, leukemia, myelodysplastic syndromes, liver hepatomas or adenomas, and other solid tumors. One quarter of aplastic anemia cases seen are FA. Death is due to **bone marrow failure.** Solid tumor cancers are increased hundreds- to thousands-fold.

Treatment **Marrow or stem cell transplantation,** androgens, corticosteroids, surgery for thumb and radial defects.

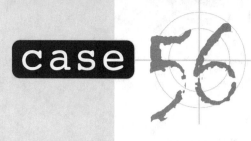

case 56

ID/CC A 10-year-old **male** is referred to a genetic evaluation clinic by his pediatrician because of **mental retardation.**

HPI His mother did not take any drugs during her pregnancy, did not suffer from any major illnesses, was seen by an obstetrician periodically, and was monitored intrapartum.

PE Patient is well developed physically with grade I mental retardation; **macrocephaly** with large jaw and ears; midsystolic click heard in mitral area; enlarged testes (macro-orchidism).

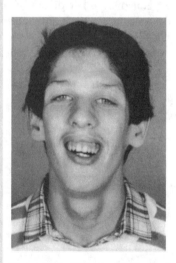

Figure 56-1. Patient exhibiting features of macrocephaly, long face, large ears, high arched palate, and prominent nasal bridge.

Labs Patient has been subjected to basic and endocrinologic lab profiles; Molecular genetics: PCR and Southern blot show marked **CGG triplet expansion** on **FMR1 gene** on long arm of X chromosome. Karyotype: **"fragile gap" at end of the long arm on X chromosome.**

111

case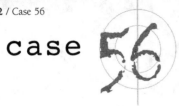

Fragile X Syndrome

Differential

Marfan Syndrome

Ehlers-Danlos Syndrome

Pervasive Developmental Disorders

Attention-Deficit/Hyperactivity Disorder

Rett Syndrome

Discussion

The **second most common cause of mental retardation** after Down's syndrome **in males** (women are carriers), Fragile X syndrome should be suspected in any male patient whose mental retardation cannot be explained by other disease processes. The disorder demonstrates genetic **anticipation** (worsening of the disorder in successive generations) owing to the expansion of **trinucleotide repeats**.

Treatment

Supportive.

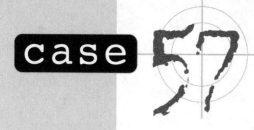

case 57

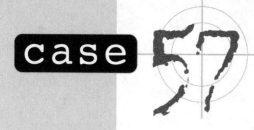

ID/CC A 2-week-old white baby is taken to a doctor because of lethargy, **feeding difficulties,** and yellowish skin (JAUNDICE).

HPI The child has been **vomiting** on and off since birth.

PE Irritability; **jaundice; cataracts; hepatomegaly;** edema.

Labs Positive on newborn screen. UA: **galactosuria;** aminoaciduria; albuminuria. **Hypoglycemia;** increased ALT and AST; elevated direct and indirect bilirubin; prolonged PT; erythrocytes have **markedly reduced galactose-1-phosphate uridyl transferase activity** and elevated galactose-1-phosphate.

Imaging US/CT: enlarged fatty liver.

Gross Pathology Early hepatomegaly and fatty change with giant cells leading to cirrhosis; gliosis of cerebral cortex, basal ganglia, and dentate nucleus of cerebellum; cataracts.

Micro Pathology Liver, eyes, and brain most severely affected by **deposits of galactose-1-phosphate and galactitol;** kidney, heart, and spleen also involved.

case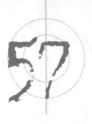

Galactosemia

Differential

Galactose Deficiency

Fructose Intolerance (fructose 1-P aldolase deficiency)

Hemochromatosis

Sepsis

Alpha 1–antitrypsin Deficiency

Discussion

Galactosemia is an **autosomal-recessive** lack of enzyme **galactose-1-phosphate uridyl transferase**; the presence of **cataracts** differentiates it from other causes of jaundice in the newborn.

Breakout Point

The Defective Enzyme in Galactosemia
Galactose-1-phosphate uridyl transferase catalyzes: **galactose-1-phosphate+UDP glucose → UDP galactose+glucose-1-phosphate.**

Treatment

Limit intake of milk and other galactose- and lactose-containing foods.

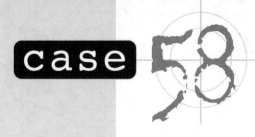

case 58

ID/CC An 11-year-old **Jewish** male presents with weakness, **epistaxis,** and a left-sided abdominal mass.

HPI He has a history of **bruising easily** and sustaining fractures following minimal trauma.

PE Mental retardation; multiple **purpuric patches;** skin pigmentation; mild hepatomegaly; **massive spleno-megaly;** marked pallor; no lymphadenopathy or icterus.

Labs CBC: normocytic, normochromic anemia; thrombocytopenia; low normal WBC count. LFTs normal; bone marrow biopsy characteristic; isolated WBCs demonstrate **reduced acid beta-glucosidase** activity; elevated serum acid phosphatase.

Imaging XR: spine: biconcave (H-shaped) vertebral bodies. XR: knee: Erlenmeyer flask deformity of distal femur; osteopenia. CT/US: enlarged spleen with multiple nodules.

Micro Pathology Bone marrow biopsy shows myelophthisis; replaced by cells 20–100 μm in size; characteristic **"wrinkled tissue paper" cytoplasm** due to intracytoplasmic glucocerebroside deposition; PAS stain positive.

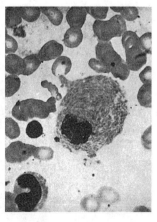

Figure 58-1. Wrinkled tissue paper cytoplasm.

115

case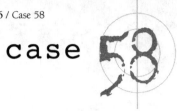

Gaucher Disease

Differential

Niemann-Pick Disease

Thalassemia

Acute Lymphocytic Leukemia

Mucopolysaccharidoses

Discussion

Gaucher disease is a lipid storage disease inherited in an **autosomal-recessive** manner and results in a **deficiency of acid beta-glucocerebrosidase** with **accumulation of glucosyl-ceramide** in bone marrow, spleen, and liver, leading to **pancytopenia.**

Treatment

Symptomatic, enzyme replacement therapy with recombinant beta-glucocerebrosidase (Imiglucerase), glucosylceramide synthase inhibitor (Miglustat), splenectomy.

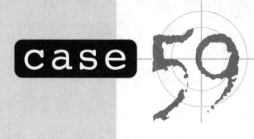

case 59

GENETICS

ID/CC A 5-month-old male is brought to the doctor because of frequent nausea, **vomiting,** night sweats, tremors, and **lethargy.**

HPI When the patient was exclusively breast fed (i.e., during the initial four months after birth), he was asymptomatic; the **onset of symptoms coincided with** the occasional **addition of fruit juices** to the baby's diet.

PE Lazy-looking, slightly **jaundiced** baby; mild growth retardation; **hepatomegaly.**

Labs **Marked hypoglycemia; fructosemia.** ABGs: metabolic acidosis. UA: fructosuria; urine test for reducing sugar positive; dipstick for glucose negative; fructose tolerance test not advisable (may cause severe hypoglycemia).

Micro Pathology Liver biopsy reveals **low aldolase B activity** (confirmatory test).

case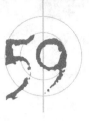

Hereditary Fructose Intolerance

Differential

Metabolic Acidosis

Lactose Intolerance

Failure to Thrive

Reye Syndrome

Discussion

Any food containing fructose or sucrose (fructose + glucose) may cause symptoms in patients with fructose intolerance, an **autosomal-recessive deficiency of aldolase B,** resulting in accumulation of fructose-1-phosphate within liver cells. Aldolase B is an essential enzyme in the process of gluconeogenesis; it is reversible, and central to glycolysis forming the triose phosphates thus inhibiting glycolysis, gluconeogenesis, and glycogenolysis. If long-standing, it may lead to cirrhosis and kidney failure. Differential diagnosis is galactosemia.

Breakout Point

> **The deficiency in hereditary fructose intolerance is:**
>
> **aldolase B** that catalyzes a 6 carbon compound into 3 carbon compounds:
>
> fructose-1-phosphate → glyceraldehyde + dihydroxyacetone phosphate

Treatment

Return to breast feeding as sole food; avoid fruit juices, fruits, and sweets containing fructose, sucrose, or sorbitol; avoid prolonged fasting.

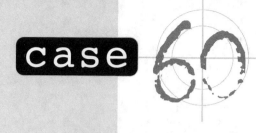

case 60

ID/CC A 9-year-old male is referred to the pediatric clinic because of progressive **mental retardation, diminished visual acuity,** and **bone deformity** in the thorax.

HPI The boy was born in Malaysia and never had any prenatal screening.

PE Tall and thin with elongated limbs (Marfanoid appearance); fine hair; **abnormally long fingers** (ARACHNODACTYLY); **pectus excavatum; lenticular dislocation** (ECTOPIA LENTIS); malar flush; high-arched palate; genu valgum ("knock-knees"); cardiovascular exam normal.

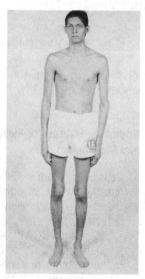

Figure 60-1. Patient presentation

Labs Increased plasma methionine and homocystine; positive cyanidenitroprusside urine test; deficient cystathionine beta-synthase activity upon liver biopsy.

Imaging XR: generalized **osteoporosis.**

Micro Pathology Brain gliosis; arterial intimal thickening without lipid deposition; degeneration of zonular ligaments of lens.

119

case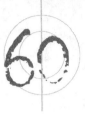

Homocystinuria

Differential

Thrombophlebitis

Marfan Syndrome

Discussion

Homocystinuria is an autosomal-recessive **defect of methionine metabolism** caused by a **deficiency of cystathionine synthase** in liver cells with accumulation of **homocystine.** Major arterial and venous **thromboses** are a constant threat because of vessel wall changes and increased platelet adhesiveness due to the toxicity of homocystine to the vascular endothelium.

Treatment

High-dose pyridoxine (cofactor for cystathionine synthetase; effective only in some forms of disease); anti-homocystinuric as a methyl donor (betaine); B12 (cyanocobalamin); methionine-restricted diet; cysteine and folate supplements.

Breakout Point

Additional Causes for Elevated Homocysteine and Methionine:

1. Defect in vitamin B-12 synthesis from remethylation of homocysteine to methionine.
2. Defect in *N*-5,10-methylenetetrahydrofolate reductase.
3. Type 2 vitamin B-12 metabolic defect.
4. Intestinal malabsorption of vitamin B12.
5. Homocystinuria responsive to vitamin B12 (type E cobalamin [cbl]).
6. Transcobalamin II deficiency.
7. Methylcobalamin deficiency with type G cbl.

case 61

ID/CC A 6-year-old **male** is sent to the audiometry clinic by his pediatrician for an evaluation of **deafness**.

His teachers note that he has not been paying attention at school and add that his academic performance has suffered as a result. His brother had similar problems two years previously.

PE **Coarse facies and large tongue;** short stature; **corneas clear;** dimpled skin in back of arms and thighs; no gibbus (acute-angle kyphosis) present; nonpainful nodular lesions on left scapular area; stiffening of joints; **deafness.**

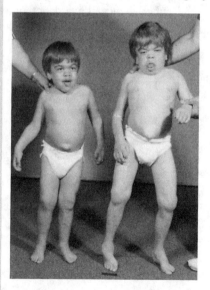

Figure 61-1. Patient and older brother at presentation.

Labs UA: **increased urinary heparan sulfate and dermatan sulfate.** Decreased iduronate sulfatase activity in WBCs.

Imaging Metacarpal thickening with tapering at ends.

Micro Pathology Metachromatic granules (REILLY BODIES) in bone marrow leukocytes; amniotic fluid culture during pregnancy may detect abnormality.

121

case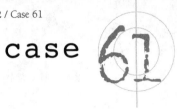

Hunter Disease

Differential

Hurler Syndrome

Scheie Syndrome

Sanfilippo Syndrome

Sly Disease

Discussion

Hunter disease, or type II mucopolysaccharidosis, is an **X-linked recessive lysosomal storage disease** and is less severe than Hurler syndrome (type I). Hunter disease can be differentiated from Hurler syndrome in that it features no corneal opacities and either no mental retardation or less severe retardation than that found in Hurler; however, deafness is present. This disease is caused by a **deficiency of iduronosulfate 2-sulfatase.**

Treatment

Supportive.

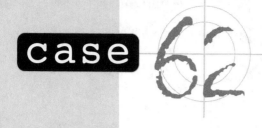

ID/CC A **2-year-old** white male is brought to the ophthalmologist for an evaluation of **eye clouding**.

HPI The child has a physical and **mental disability** very similar to that of his older **brother**.

PE **Short stature**; very **coarse, elongated facial features** (GARGOYLISM); **bilateral corneal opacities**; retinal degeneration and papilledema; saddle nose deformity; systolic murmur in second right intercostal space; **enlarged heart, liver, and spleen; kyphoscoliosis** with lumbar gibbus (acute angle kyphosis); stiff, immobile, and contracted large joints.

Labs Dermatan sulfate and heparan sulfate in urine; **alpha-L-iduronidase deficiency in WBCs**.

Imaging XR: dolichocephaly; increased diameter of sella turcica; deformation of vertebral bodies with scoliosis and kyphosis.

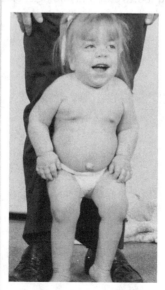

Figure 62-1. Note the characteristic facies and posture.

123

case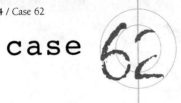

Hurler Disease

Differential

Hunter Syndrome
Schie Syndrome
Sanfilippo Syndrome
Morquio Syndrome
Maroteaux-Lamy Syndrome

Discussion

Also known as gargoylism, Hurler syndrome is the most common of the mucopolysaccharidoses (TYPE I). It is **autosomal recessive** and is caused by a **deficiency of alpha-L-iduronidase** degrading its **substrates heparin sulfate and dermatan sulfate**. Death usually occurs by 6 to 10 years of age, usually secondary to cardiovascular complications.

Treatment

Enzyme replacement therapy with recombinant alpha-L-iduronidase (Laronidase) provides some symptomatic relief and delays ongoing symptoms. Supportive ophthalmologic, skeletal, and cardiovascular treatment. Consider bone marrow transplant.

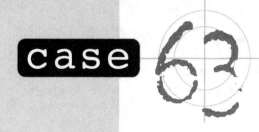

ID/CC A 19-year-old male visits his family physician because he is **embarrassed at having large breasts**.

HPI He also complains of frequent headaches and **impotence**.

PE **Tall, eunuchoid** body habitus; mild mental retardation; testes small and firm; breast enlargement (GYNECOMASTIA); female distribution of hair.

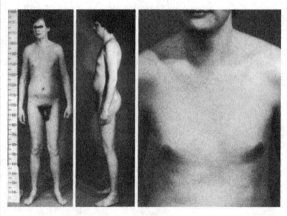

Figure 63-1. Patient exhibiting eunuchoid habitus, gynecomastia, hypogonadism, and long limbs.

Labs High serum FSH, LH, and estradiol; low serum testosterone. UA: high FSH and LH. Karyotype: XXY.

Imaging XR: delayed physeal closure; short fourth metacarpal.

Gross Pathology Testicular atrophy.

Micro Pathology **Testicular fibrosis and hyalinization; lack of spermatogenesis;** Leydig's interstitial cells scarce and have foamy cytoplasmic change; **female sex chromatin bodies** (BARR BODIES) in cells.

case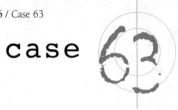

Klinefelter Syndrome

Differential

Hypogonadism
Fragile X Syndrome
Marfan Syndrome
Kallman Syndrome
46, XX Male
Infertility

Discussion

Also known as **testicular dysgenesis**, Klinefelter syndrome is the most common cause of male hypogonadism. Alteration is due to the presence of three sex chromosomes (karyotype 47, XXY).

Treatment

Androgen replacement therapy (testosterone).

case 64

ID/CC   A **5-month-old** child is brought to the pediatrician because of **growth retardation** and **difficulty feeding.**

HPI   His parents note that the child has been **irritable** and "stiff" (SPASTICITY).

PE   VS: normal. PE: patient **underdeveloped** for age; **reflexes hyperactive;** paravertebral muscles and hamstrings tense (RIGIDITY); maternal milk **sucking reflex weak** and punctuated by periods of regurgitation.

Labs   Basic lab work within normal limits. LP: increased protein in CSF. Low beta-galactosidase activity in leukocytes.

Imaging CT head without contrast: Lesions of increased density adjacent to the lateral ventricles.

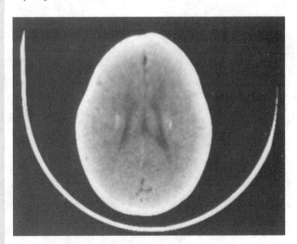

Figure 64-1. Nonenhanced brain CT scan.

Gross Pathology   Axonal and white-matter cerebral, cerebellar, and basal ganglia **demyelination.**

Micro Pathology   Basophilic perivascular multinucleated globoid cells with cytoplasmic inclusion bodies consisting of cerebroside (globoid cells).

127

case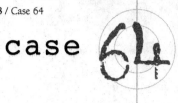

Krabbe Disease

Differential

Gaucher Disease

Niemann-Pick Disease

GM2 Gangliosidoses

Metachromatic Leukodystrophy

Canavan Disease

Discussion

Also called **globoid leukodystrophy,** Krabbe disease is an **autosomal-recessive,** familial genetic disorder characterized by a **deficiency of galactosylceramide beta-galactosidase.**

Treatment

Poor prognosis, with death usually occurring rapidly.

case

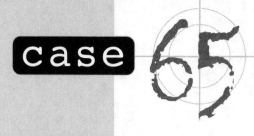

ID/CC A 2-year-old **male** is brought to the pediatrician by his mother because of repeated, **self-mutilating biting of his fingers and lips;** the patient's mother has also noticed abundant, **orange-colored "sand"** (uric acid crystals) **in the child's diapers.**

HPI The mother reports that some months ago the child's urine was red, but she took no action at the time.

PE Poor head control, difficulty walking, and difficulty maintaining an erect, seated position; **choreoathetoid movements,** spasticity, and **hyperreflexia** on neurologic exam.

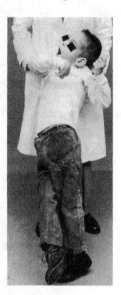

Figure 65-1. Choreoathetosis of upper extremities and scissoring of lower extremities.

Labs **Hyperuricemia** (>10 mg/dL). UA: crystalluria; microscopic hematuria (due to renal calculi). Low HGPRT activity in blood and fibroblasts.

Imaging XR: irregular amputation of several fingers.

129

case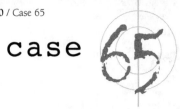

Lesch–Nyhan Syndrome

Differential

Childhood Chorea

Cerebral Palsy

Mental Retardation

Dystonia

Discussion

Lesch–Nyhan syndrome is an **X-linked recessive** metabolic disease resulting from a deficiency of an enzyme of purine metabolism, **hypoxanthine-guanine phosphoribosyl transferase (HGPRT).** If left untreated, patients develop full-blown **gouty arthritis** and urate nephropathy as well as subcutaneous tophaceous deposits. Neurological problems are present, and compulsive, uncontrollable destructive behavior is typical of the disorder. Prenatal diagnosis is possible.

Treatment

Uricosuric agents (Allopurinol). Removal of primary teeth to prevent self-injury; hydration to prevent nephrolithiasis; antispasmodics and benzodiazepines for neurologic symptoms.

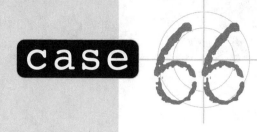

case 66

ID/CC A **5-day-old** Mennonite male presents with **seizures**, difficulty feeding, and vomiting; his mother reports a **peculiar, maple-sugar-like odor on his diapers.**

HPI His mother had an unremarkable full-term vaginal delivery.

PE VS: no fever. PE: full-term neonate with irregular respirations, **muscular rigidity** (SPASTICITY), and obtunded sensorium; fundus normal; peculiar odor in urine and sweat; when child's head support (hand) is suddenly withdrawn in supine position, patient fails to react with normal extension-abduction followed by flexion and adduction of arms (ABSENCE OF MORO REFLEX).

Labs **Hypoglycemia.** ABGs: metabolic acidosis. **Marked elevation in blood and urine levels of the branched chain amino acids (and their keto acids): leucine, isoleucine, and valine** as well as decreased levels of alanine, threonine, and serine.

Gross Pathology Edema of brain with gliosis and white matter **demyelination.**

case 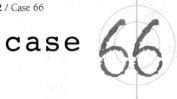 66

Maple Syrup Urine Disease

Differential

Hydroxyprolinemia
Isovaleric Acidemia
Propionic Acidemia
Non-ketotic Hyperglycemia

Discussion

Maple syrup urine disease is an **autosomal-recessive** branched-chain alpha-ketoaciduria that results from defective oxidative decarboxylation of the branched-chain alpha-ketoacids. This decarboxylation is accomplished by an enzyme complex (**α-ketodehydrogenase**) using thiamine as a coenzyme. A **deficiency** of this enzyme system in the disease causes urine to have the characteristic maple syrup odor and causes CNS symptoms in the first few weeks of life. Leucine causes the primary neuropathy by crossing the blood-brain barrier and forms glutamate (an excitatory neurotransmitter) and glutamine.

Treatment

Restricting intake of branched-chain amino acids from diet; thiamine supplementation.

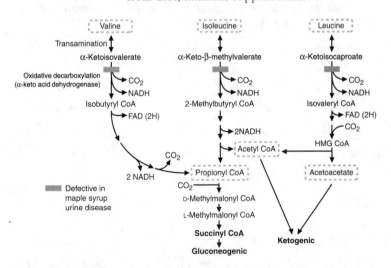

Figure 66-1. Maple syrup urine disease: defect in the degradation of branched chain amino acids.

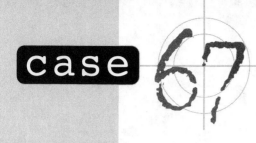

ID/CC	A 3-year-old white male is brought to the pediatrician because of **increasing difficulty walking** due to **spasticity**.
HPI	The child had been developing normally up to now, and his medical history is unremarkable.
PE	**Difficulty climbing stairs; ataxia; wide-based gait;** extensor plantar response and hyperreflexia.
Labs	Decreased leukocyte arylsulfatase A enzyme activity. UA: **elevated sulfatide** levels. LP: increased protein in CSF (vs. cerebral palsy). Decreased peripheral nerve conduction velocity.
Imaging	MR: brain: demyelination.
Gross Pathology	Generalized **demyelination** (due to deficiency of arylsulfatase A interfering with normal metabolism of myelin lipids) with gliosis.
Micro Pathology	Toluidine blue staining shows brownish (METACHRO-MATIC) granules in oligodendrocytes and neurons of globus pallidus, thalamus, and dentate nucleus.

case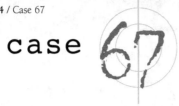

Metachromatic Leukodystrophy

Differential

Krabbe Disease

Cerebral Palsy

Schizophrenia

X-linked Adrenoleukodystrophy

Discussion

Metachromatic leukodystrophy is a lysosomal storage disease with an **autosomal-recessive** mode of inheritance involved in **sphingolipid metabolism** that is due to a **deficiency in the enzyme arylsulfatase A** with accumulation of sulfated glycolipids (sulfatides) in the central and peripheral nervous system as well as in the kidneys. Intrauterine diagnosis is possible.

Treatment

No effective treatment. Poor prognosis; patients become invalids within a few years and die within five years of the onset of symptoms.

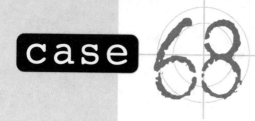
ID/CC An 11-month-old **Jewish** male of **Ashkenazi** descent presents with globally delayed development and **diminished visual acuity.**

HPI His parents feel that the baby is not acquiring new skills and that existing ones are regressing. They also feel that their child cannot see or hear properly.

PE **Hepatosplenomegaly; cherry-red spot on macula** on funduscopy; malnourished infant with protuberant abdomen; global developmental delay; hypoacusis.

Labs CBC: mild normochromic, normocytic anemia. Decreased leukocyte **sphingomyelinase** activity.

Micro Pathology Bone marrow biopsy reveals sphingomyelinase deficiency in cultured skin fibroblasts; characteristic "foam cells" containing sphingomyelin and cholesterol.

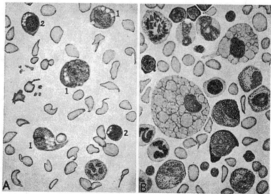

Figure 68-1. Large foam cell from peripheral blood smear.

case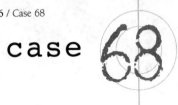

Niemann–Pick Disease

Differential

Gaucher Disease

GM1 Gangliosidosis

Wilson Disease

Maple Syrup Urine Disease

Alpha-Antitrypsin Deficiency

Discussion

Niemann–Pick disease is an **autosomal-recessive deficiency of acid sphingomyelinase** with **accumulation of sphingomyelin** (a ceramide phospholipid) **in lysosomes** of monocyte/macrophage system, histiocytes in the brain, bone marrow, spleen, and liver.

Treatment

No treatment available. Carries a poor prognosis, with death occurring within a few years of birth.

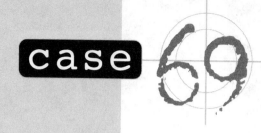

ID/CC A 2-year-old female is referred to a pediatric clinic for evaluation of **lethargy, weakness, and persistent anemia** that has been **unresponsive to treatment with vitamin B$_{12}$, folic acid,** iron, and vitamin C.

HPI She is the third-born child of a healthy white couple; her mother had an uneventful pregnancy and a eutopic delivery. Both brothers are healthy.

PE **Low weight and height** for age; **marked pallor;** flaccidity and lethargy; **sleepiness.** No focal neurologic signs; lungs clear; heart sound with slight aortic systolic ejection murmur (due to anemia); abdomen soft; no masses; no hepatomegaly; spleen barely palpable; no lymphadenopathy.

Labs CBC: **megaloblastic anemia;** elevated mean corpuscular volume. UA: increased orotic acid excretion with formation of **orotic acid crystals.**

case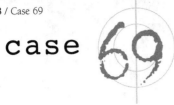

Orotic Aciduria

Differential | Type II Orotic Aciduria
Methylmalonic Academia
Hepatic Encephalopathy
Carbamoyl Phosphate Synthetase Deficiency
Ornithine Transcarbamylase Deficiency

Discussion | Orotic aciduria is an **autosomal-recessive disorder of pyrimidine synthesis**; it is caused by a deficiency of the enzyme complex **orotidylic pyrophosphorylase-orotidylic decarboxylase** with resultant megaloblastic anemia due to impaired synthesis of nucleic acids necessary for hematopoiesis.

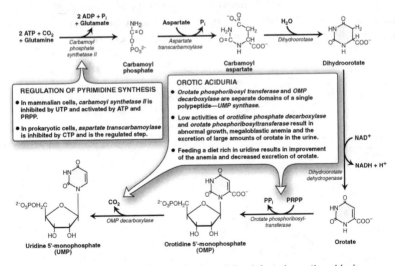

Figure 69-1. De novo pyrimidine synthesis and the defects in orotic aciduria.

Treatment | Administration of **uridine** and cytidine.

case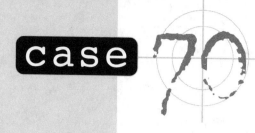

ID/CC A 5-year-old white male is brought to the emergency room with a fracture of his right forearm that he sustained after falling off a couch.

HPI This is the **fifth bone fracture** that the child has sustained **in the past 2 years.**

PE **Bluish sclera;** right leg and right arm slightly deformed from poor healing of past fractures; mild **kyphosis and scoliosis** of thoracic spine; **hypotonia and laxity** of right leg and arm; **partial conduction deafness** in both ears.

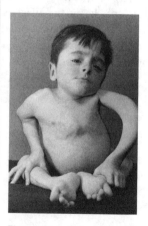

Figure 70-1. Bony deformities secondary to multiple fractures following minor trauma.

Imaging XR: fracture of radius and ulna with evidence of osteopenia.

Micro Pathology **Marked thinning of bone cortices** (EGGSHELL CORTEX) and rarefaction of trabeculae (due to **abnormal synthesis of type I collagen**); abnormal softening of tooth enamel.

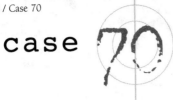

case

Osteogenesis Imperfecta

Differential

Physical Child Abuse
Congenital Hypophosphatasia
Steroid Induced Osteoporosis
Idiopathic Juvenile Osteoporosis

Discussion

Also called brittle bone disease, osteogenesis imperfecta is an **autosomal-dominant** disorder of type I collagen synthesis in which there is deficient ossification due to inadequate osteoid formation. Defects can be manifested by quality (abnormal Type I collagen produced) or quantity (decrease in Type I collagen production). It can be diagnosed *in utero* by DNA analysis and prenatal ultrasound. Type I osteogenesis imperfecta is the most common and has an onset in infancy. Hearing loss in middle age common.

Treatment

Supportive. If severe osteopenia and repeated fractures, Pamidronate may increase bone mineral density and reduce fractures.

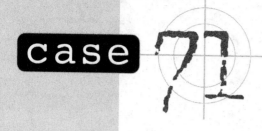

case 71

ID/CC   A 3-year-old male of Turkish descent presents with progressive **mental retardation, vomiting,** and **hyperactivity** with purposeless movements.

HPI   The child developed normally for the first 2 to 3 months. He is fairer than his siblings and, unlike them, has blue eyes. He was born outside the United States and did not undergo any screening for congenital disorders.

PE   Child is **blond with blue eyes, perspires** heavily, is mentally retarded, and has **peculiar "mousy" odor; hypertonia** with hyperactive deep tendon reflexes on neurologic exam.

Labs   Guthrie test (bacterial inhibition assay method) positive (due to **increased blood phenylalanine levels**); increased urinary phenylpyruvic and ortho-hydroxyphenylacetic acid; **normal concentration of tetrahydrobiopterin.**

Imaging   XR: delayed bone age. MRI: areas of demyelination

case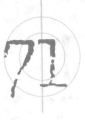

Phenylketonuria (PKU)

Differential | Hyperphenylalaninemia
Tyrosinemia
Tetrahydrobiopterin Deficiency

Discussion | PKU is an **autosomal-recessive disorder** caused by a **deficiency of the enzyme phenylalanine hydroxylase** that metabolizes phenylalanine. A neonatal screening program for the detection of PKU is in effect throughout the United States. If maternal levels of phenylalanine are high, growth and mental retardation, microcephaly, and congenital heart defects can result. Among children of women with untreated PKU, the incidence of mental retardation can be as high as 90%.

L-Phenylalanine

PKU
Phenylalanine hydroxylase

Tetrahydrobiopterin + O_2

Dihydrobiopterin + H_2O

L-Tyrosine

Figure 71-1. A deficiency in phenylalanine hydroxylase results in phenylketonuria.

Treatment | Diet formulas low in phenylalanine. Avoid aspartame. **Tyrosine supplementation.**

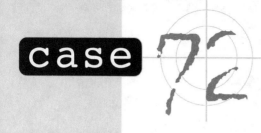

case 72

ID/CC A 7-year-old female presents with anxiety, **dizziness, sweating,** and nausea **following** brief episodes of **exercise.**

HPI These symptoms are **relieved by eating** and do not occur if the patient is frequently fed small meals.

PE Physical exam unremarkable.

Labs **Hypoglycemia** following brief fasting; alanine fails to increase blood sugar; fructose or glycerol administration restores blood glucose to normal. **Lactic acidosis.**

Micro Pathology Liver biopsy for enzyme assays reveals deficiency of phosphoenolpyruvate carboxykinase, an enzyme of gluconeogenesis; **no excess glycogen storage** revealed.

case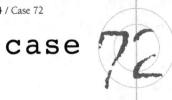

Phosphoenolpyruvate Carboxykinase Deficiency

Differential | Pyruvate Carboxylase Deficiency
Pyruvate Dehydrogenase Deficiency
Fumerase Deficiency
Leigh Encephalopathy

Discussion | Phosphoenolpyruvate carboxykinase (PEPCK) deficiency **prevents conversion of pyruvate to phosphoenolpyruvate.** This deficiency interferes with gluconeogenesis from 3-carbon precursors (e.g., alanine) that enter the gluconeogenetic pathway at or below the pyruvate level.

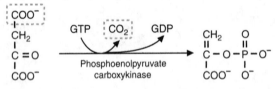

Figure 72-1. Conversion of oxaloacetate to phosphoenolpyruvate by PEPCK.

Treatment | Frequent small meals to prevent episodes of hypoglycemia.

case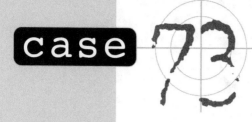

ID/CC A **6-month-old white** child is brought to the pediatrician because of **failure to gain weight,** increasing **weakness,** insufficient strength to breast feed, and **lethargy.**

HPI He is the second-born son of a healthy white couple; his mother's pregnancy and delivery were uneventful.

PE Mild cyanosis; shallow respirations; increase in size of tongue (MACROGLOSSIA); moderate hepatomegaly; **significant generalized muscular flaccidity.**

Labs CBC: normal. Lytes: normal. **Glucose,** BUN, creatinine **normal, creatine kinase 5x normal,** aspartate aminotransferase high. ECG: **short P-R; wide QRS; left-axis deviation.**

Imaging CXR: **extreme cardiomegaly** and congestive heart failure. Echo: cardiomegaly with biventricular thickening and outflow tract obstruction.

Gross Pathology Significant increase in size and weight of heart (up to five times normal); to lesser extent, hepatomegaly.

Micro Pathology Extensive intracytoplasmic and lysosomal deposition of glycogen on myocardial fibers as well as in striated muscle fibers, kidney, and liver.

case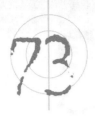

Pompe Disease

Differential

Noonan Syndrome
Spinal Muscular Atrophy
Werdnig-Hoffman Disease
Carnitine Deficiency
Mitochondrial Disorders
Myocarditis

Discussion

Pompe disease is also a **type II glycogen storage disease** (generalized). This fatal disorder is caused by an **autosomal-recessive deficiency in the lysosomal hydrolase** (only glycogenolysis with lysosomal involvement) **alpha-1,4-glucosidase** (ACID MALTASE), with resulting accumulation of structurally normal glycogen in the heart, muscle, kidney, and liver. This case illustrates the infantile form.

Breakout Point

> ### Mutations of Alpha-1,4-glucosidase Can Result In:
>
> Infantile form with NO enzyme activity.
> Normal amount of enzyme with reduced activity (affinity) for glycogen.
> Reduced amount of enzyme, but that which remains has normal activity.

Treatment

Poor prognosis; associated with early death from **cardiopulmonary failure.** In 2006, enzyme replacement therapy was introduced with recombinant human alpha-glucosidase (Aglucosidase alfa).

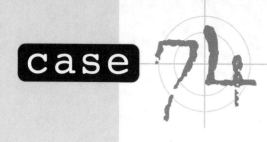

case 74

ID/CC A 40-year-old **male** visits his family doctor because of a **chronic, recurrent rash** on his hands, face, and other **sun-exposed areas**; the patient's **urine turns dark brown-black if left standing**, and he has noticed that recurrences coincide with **alcohol intake**.

HPI He reports having used **hexachlorobenzene** (halogenated aromatic hydrocarbons) **as a pesticide** for some years.

PE Skin erythema with **vesicles and bullae on sun-exposed areas**; skin at these sites is friable and shows presence of whitish plaques ("MILIA") (due to photosensitizing effect of uroporphyrin); skin of face also shows hypertrichosis and hyperpigmentation.

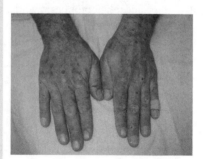

Figure 74-1. Skin eruptions in a patient.

Labs Watson–Schwartz test negative. UA: **urine fluorescent; markedly elevated urinary uroporphyrin levels; slightly elevated urinary coproporphyrin levels.** Elevated fecal isocoproporphyrin; **elevated transferrin, serum, and hepatic iron;** elevated serum transaminases.

Gross Pathology Liver shows siderosis, bullae, fibrosis, and inflammatory changes.

Micro Pathology Skin biopsy demonstrates iron deposits, intense porphyrin fluorescence, and long, thin cytoplasmic inclusions.

case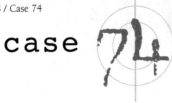

Porphyria Cutanea Tarda

Differential

Epidermolysis Bullosa
Erythropoietic Porphyria
Lupus Erythromatosis
Variegated Pophyria

Discussion

Porphyria cutanea tarda (PCT), the most common porphyria, in contrast to other hepatic porphyrias, is more common among men than women. Exposure to PCT is caused by partial loss of activity of **hepatic uroporphyrinogen decarboxylase;** lesions are caused by overproduction and excretion of uroporphyrin. Other causes are exposure to hepatitis viruses (A, B, or C), HIV, estrogen, or hemochromatosis genes.

Treatment

Repeated phlebotomies; avoidance of sunlight, alcohol, iron, and estrogens. Low dose antimalarials (Chloroquine) to bind porphyrins, then excrete; stimulate bone marrow (Epoetin alfa) if phlebotomies are contraindicated.

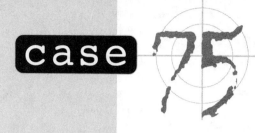

ID/CC A 5-year-old girl is referred to a pediatric hematologist for an evaluation of chronic **anemia that has been unresponsive to nutritional supplementation.**

HPI Both parents are clinically normal and are **first cousins.** The patient has no history of passage of dark-colored urine or recurrent infections.

PE Low weight and height for age; pallor; mild **jaundice;** spleen barely palpable; liver not enlarged.

Labs CBC/PBS: **anemia; markedly increased reticulocyte count;** peripheral blood reveals macro-ovalocytosis with a few acanthocytes; no sickle cells or sphero-cytes seen but shrunken RBCs. Hyper-bilirubinemia (primarily unconjugated). UA: urinary hemosiderin present.

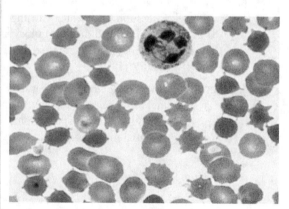

Figure 75-1. Acanthocytic red blood cells.

case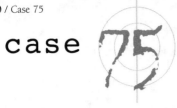

Pyruvate Kinase Deficiency

Differential

Carnitine Deficiency

Glycogen Storage Diseases

Hemoglobin H Disease

Pyruvate Carboxylase Deficiency

Thalassemia Minor

Discussion

Pyruvate kinase (PK) deficiency, one of the most common erythrocytic enzyme defects, is inherited as an **autosomal-recessive** trait and usually produces mild symptoms (hemolytic anemia); **2,3-diphosphoglycerate accumulates,** shifting the hemoglobin-oxygen dissociation curve to the right (due to reduced affinity of RBCs for oxygen). The disturbance in the cell membrane gradient by lack of adenosine triphosphate (ATP) allows loss of potassium and water causing the cell to contract, crenulate, and die. Reticulocytes can circumvent PK deficiency by utilizing oxidative phosphorylation to make ATP.

Treatment

Most do not require treatment. If severe hemolytic anemia, folic acid to prevent megaloblastic anemia. Transfusions and splenectomy (give antibiotics for potential infection prophylactically) if severe.

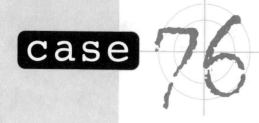

ID/CC A **6-month-old** male is brought to a pediatrician for evaluation of **listlessness**, lethargy, and **fixed gaze**.

HPI His parents are **Ashkenazi Jews**.

PE **Excessive extensor startle response to noise** (HYPERACUSIS); child is sleepy and hypotonic with poor head control and a fixed gaze; appears to have translucent skin; **cherry-red macular spot** found on funduscopic exam.

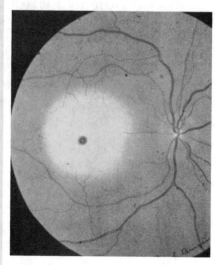

Figure 76-1. Cherry red spot on the macula.

Labs Reduced concentration of sphingomyelin in RBCs; deficient hexosaminidase A activity in serum.

Gross Pathology Diffuse gliosis; cerebral and macular degeneration; up to 50% increase in brain weight (due to deposition of sphingolipid).

Micro Pathology Neuronal swelling with cytoplasmic **deposits of gangliosides** (ZEBRA BODIES).

151

case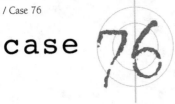

Tay–Sachs Disease

Differential

Sandhoff Disease
Gaucher Disease
GM1 Gangliosidoses

Discussion

Tay–Sachs disease (**GM2 gangliosidoses type I**), a lysosomal lipid storage disease, is an autosomal-recessive disorder of sphingolipid metabolism characterized by the **absence of the enzyme hexosaminidase A**, producing excessive storage of ganglioside GM-2 in lysosomes **restricted to the cells of the central nervous system. Ganglioside GM-2** is a glycosphingolipid with sphingosine, a long-chain basic molecule, as its backbone along with an attached sugar and a terminal N-acetylglucosamine. Prenatal diagnosis can be made at the 14th week of pregnancy.

Treatment

Poor prognosis; patients usually die of pneumonia before age 4.

case 77

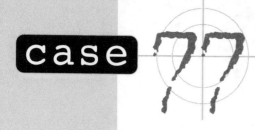

ID/CC A 5-year-old male is brought to a pediatrician for evaluation of episodes of **fatigue**, restlessness, anxiety, nausea, **lightheadedness**, vomiting, and **sweating**.

HPI The symptoms appear when he does not eat frequent meals and subside while he is eating. He also has a history of **bruising easily**.

PE Patient has **"doll-face" facies**; weight low for age; tendon xanthomas; purpuric patches over skin; **marked hepatomegaly**.

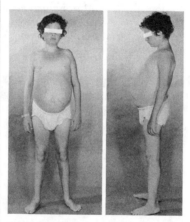

Figure 77-1. Patient exhibiting marked hepatomegaly.

Labs Lactic acidosis; hyperlipidemia; **marked increase in serum uric acid** (patient may exhibit gout symptoms); **marked hypoglycemia**; prolonged bleeding time; **lack of rise in serum glucose following** IV glucagon but striking increase in lactate; normal urinary catecholamines.

Gross Pathology **Liver and kidneys enlarged.**

Micro Pathology Hepatocytes containing variable-sized **glycogen-lipid droplets** on liver biopsy; nuclear glycogenosis seen; large glycogen deposits in kidney; skeletal and cardiac muscle not involved.

153

case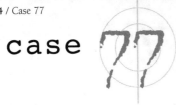

von Gierke Disease

Differential | Glycogen Storage Disease (GSD) Types II-VI
Fructose 1-P Aldolase Deficiency
Biotinidase Deficiency
Growth Hormone Deficiency
Niemann-Pick Disease

Discussion | Von Gierke disease (**Glycogen Storage Disease type I**) is **autosomal-recessive** resulting from a **deficiency of glucose-6-phosphatase** (preventing the conversion of glucose from glucose-6-phophate) and accumulation of structurally normal glycogen in the liver and kidneys. GSD Type 1b is a defect in glucose-6-phosphate **transport.**

Treatment | Frequent meals (raw cornstarch) to prevent hypoglycemia and sustain blood glucose, prophylactic iron supplementation.

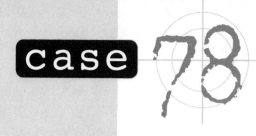

ID/CC A 3-year-old girl is brought by her parents to a dermatologist because of a recent **change in color and increase in size of a nodular lesion** on her face.

HPI She has been suffering from **excessive sensitivity to sunlight** and thus does her best to avoid the sun as much as possible.

PE Abundant **freckles** on all sun-exposed areas; **telangiectases**; areas of redness (ERYTHEMA) and hypopigmentation; **hyperkeratosis** on face and dorsum of hands; hard, nodular lesion on right cheek; no regional lymphadenopathy. Optho: **conjunctivitis.**

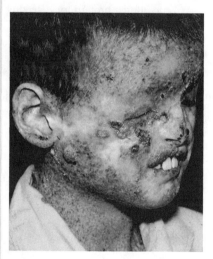

Figure 78-1. Patient presentation.

Labs Basic lab work normal.

Gross Pathology Generalized hyperpigmentation with desquamative spots on sun-exposed areas.

Micro Pathology Biopsy of cheek lesion reveals hyperkeratosis with melanin deposition; **squamous cell carcinoma.**

case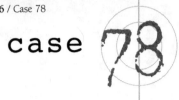

Xeroderma Pigmentosum

Differential
Cockayne Syndrome
Bloom Syndrome
Lupus Erythematosus
Hartnup Disease

Discussion
Xeroderma pigmentosum is an **autosomal-recessive** disorder that is usually manifested in childhood. It is characterized by excessive sensitivity to ultraviolet light due to **impaired nucleotide excision repair mechanism** of **ultraviolet light-damaged DNA.** UV light causes **cross linking** of pyrimidine residues in dermal fibroblasts. There are seven genes, each encoding a protein for detecting, opening the double strand, excision and repair (XPC is the most common defect). There is a marked tendency to develop **skin cancer** (squamous cell and basal cell carcinoma). Overall life expectancy reduced by about 30 years.

Treatment
Avoidance of sunlight, protection against sunlight. Surgical removal of cancer.

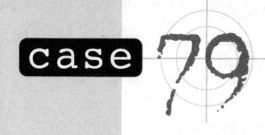

case 79

ID/CC A 20-year-old black female visits her gynecologist because she thinks she might be pregnant because of **lack of menses for the past 4 months.**

HPI She is a **pentathlon athlete** who is training to compete in her home state's tournament next fall. She is sexually active, uses the "rhythm method" for birth control, **and has never missed a menstrual period.**

PE No breast enlargement; no softening of cervix; no bluish discoloration of cervix (both presumptive signs of pregnancy); no abdominal or pelvic masses or palpable uterus; no hirsutism or virilization.

Labs Serum and urinary beta-hCG **negative for pregnancy;** serum prolactin and TSH normal; **decreased serum FSH;** no withdrawal bleeding after administration of progesterone; **normal serum androgens.**

Imaging MR, brain: normal sella and pituitary gland.

case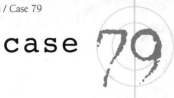

Secondary Amenorrhea

Differential | Anorexia Nervosa
Hyperthyroidism
Prolactinoma

Discussion | The **most common cause of secondary amenorrhea is pregnancy.** Primary amenorrhea is defined as the failure of menses by age 16 years. Secondary amenorrhea is cessation of menses once they have begun. Women who are involved in vigorous physical exercise and who lose weight may present with a functional gonadotropin deficit. When body weight falls to less than 15% of ideal weight, GnRH secretion from the hypothalamus is decreased, producing a secondary amenorrhea. The inhibitory effect of estrogens on bone resorption is also lost, predisposing patients to an increased risk for osteoporosis.

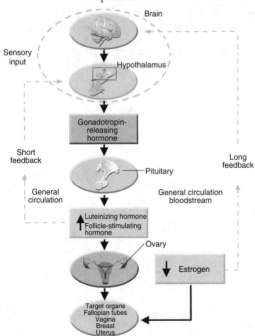

Figure 79-1. Hormonal cascade and regulation of reproduction in the female

Treatment | Advise patient to increase caloric intake, especially of fats. Oral contraceptives to prevent osteoporosis.

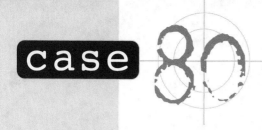
ID/CC A 62-year-old woman presents with **weakness, easy fatigability, nausea,** and **diarrhea.**

HPI She has had a long and severe course of rheumatoid arthritis for which she has been taking **methotrexate** (a folic acid antagonist).

PE VS: normal. PE: **pallor;** mild tongue inflammation (GLOSSITIS); funduscopic exam normal; chest sounds within normal limits; abdomen shows no hepatosplenomegaly; no lymphadenopathy.

Labs CBC: **hypersegmented PMNs** (>5 to 7 lobes); **macrocytic RBCs** (mean corpuscular volume >100); **vitamin B$_{12}$ level normal.**

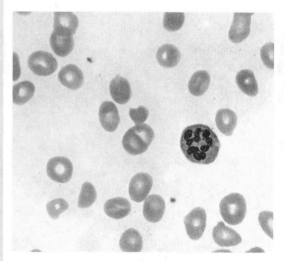

Figure 80-1. Macrocytic RBCs and hypersegmented PMNs.

HEMATOLOGY

case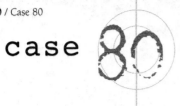

Folate Deficiency Anemia

Differential
Pernicious Anemia
Fanconi Syndrome
Vitamin B$_{12}$ Deficiency
Malabsorptive Syndromes
Intestinal Protozaol Disease
Celiac Sprue

Discussion
Folic acid is found mainly in green leaves and is important for the **synthesis of DNA and RNA**. It also acts as a coenzyme for 1-carbon transfer and is involved in **methylation reactions.** Deficiency is associated with alcoholism, pregnancy (MEGALOBLASTIC ANEMIA OF PREGNANCY), dietary deficiencies, and drugs such as TMP-SMX, methotrexate, phenytoin, and proguanil.

Treatment
Folic acid supplementation.

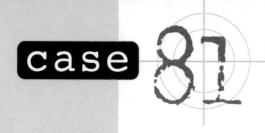

case 87

ID/CC	A 31-year-old **black male** who works as a Peace Corps volunteer in Ghana visits his medical officer complaining of extreme **weakness and fatigue;** he also complains of a **yellowing of his skin** and **slight fever.**
HPI	He was prescribed **primaquine** for radical treatment of malaria (due to *Plasmodium vivax*).
PE	VS: tachycardia (HR 95). PE: mild jaundice; circumoral and nail bed **pallor;** no hepatosplenomegaly; remainder of PE normal.
Labs	**Elevated indirect bilirubin.** CBC/PBS: **low hemoglobin and hematocrit** (9.3/33) with reticulocytosis; **spherocytes** in peripheral blood smear. Elevated LDH; reduced haptoglobin; **Heinz bodies** (precipitated hemoglobin) in RBCs; UA: hemoglobinuria.

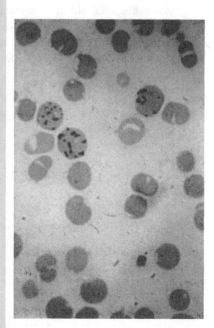

Figure 81-1. Heinz bodies in erythrocytes.

HEMATOLOGY

161

case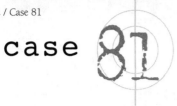

Glucose-6-Phosphate Dehydrogenase Deficiency

Differential

Sickle Cell Anemia

Hemolytic Anemia

Hereditary Spherocytosis

Discussion

Glucose-6-phosphate dehydrogenase (G6PD) deficiency is the most common enzymopathy producing clinical symptoms, and is an **X-linked recessive** disorder seen in about 15% of American black males (and 400 million people worldwide) and has the evolutionary advantage of protecting against malaria. With infections or exposure to certain drugs (e.g., sulfa drugs, antimalarials, nitrofurantoin), patients deficient in G6PD present with a **hemolytic anemia due to increased RBC sensitivity to oxidant damage.** G6PD is the rate-limiting enzyme in the Hexose Monophosphate shunt that catalyzes **oxidation** of glucose-6-phosphate $\rightarrow$ 6-phosphogluconate and concomitantly **reduces** the oxidized form of nicotinamide adenine dinucleotide phosphate NADP+ $\rightarrow$ NADPH.

Treatment

Withdrawal of the offending drug that precipitated the crisis (oxidant drugs, e.g., antimalarials, sulfonamides, ciprofloxacin niridazole, nitrofurantoin, fava beans for those of Mediterranean descent). Vigorous hydration is required to protect against renal failure secondary to hemoglobinuria.

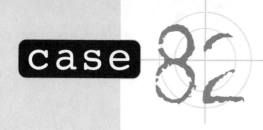

ID/CC A 7-year-old male is brought to the emergency room because of weakness and the **spontaneous appearance** of painful swelling of both knee joints (due to hemarthrosis) as well as black, tarry stools (GI bleeding).

HPI The child has a **history of prolonged bleeding following minor injuries.** His maternal uncle died of a "bleeding disorder."

PE Pallor; swollen, erythematous, tender knee joints with blood accumulation in synovial capsule (HEMARTHROSIS); numerous **bruises** seen at areas of minimal repeated trauma.

Labs Bleeding time and PT normal; **prolonged PTT;** reduced levels of factor VIII on immunoassay; **negative factor VIII inhibitors;** synovial fluid hemorrhagic.

Imaging XR: bilateral knee effusions.

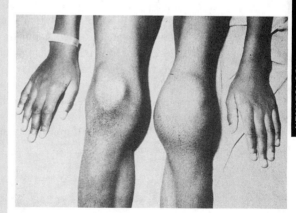

Figure 82-1. Acute hemarthrosis and its sequelae in a patient.

HEMATOLOGY

Micro Pathology Synovium may show hyperplasia with hemosiderin in synovial macrophages.

163

case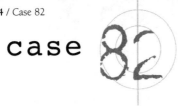

Hemophilia

Differential

Factor V, VII, X, XI Deficiencies

Glanzmann Thrombasthenia

von Willebrand Disease

Discussion

The case presented, Hemophilia A, the "classic" form, is an **X-linked recessive disorder** that is manifested by bleeding and is due to a **deficiency in coagulation factor VIII**. Hemophilia B, Christmas disease, a consequence of a congenital deficiency of coagulation factor IX, is also an X-linked recessive disorder. The concentration of these factors predicts the severity of the disease.

Treatment

Nonpharmacologic therapy involves patient education, **avoidance of contact sports**, **avoidance of aspirin** and other **NSAIDs** (due to antiplatelet aggregating effect), **orthopedic evaluation** and physical therapy, and **hepatitis vaccination**. **Recombinant factor VIII supplementation** is effective in controlling spontaneous and traumatic hemorrhage with lower risk of viral contamination. **Desmopressin**, raising endogenous levels, may be used prophylactically in patients with mild hemophilia, prior to minor surgical procedures. Antifibrinolytics (**Aminocaproic acid or Tranexamic acid**), may be used to stop bleeding that is unresponsive to factor VIII or desmopressin.

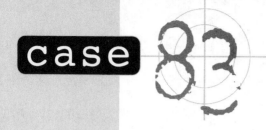

case 83

ID/CC A 9-month-old infant is brought to the pediatrician because of **jaundice**, lethargy, and **easy fatigability**.

HPI The parents of the child are immigrants of **northern European origin**.

PE Pallor; mild jaundice; palpable **splenomegaly**.

Labs CBC/PBS: microcytic **anemia**; small, **rounded**, dark RBCs lacking central pallor (SPHEROCYTES); negative Coombs test. **Elevated indirect bilirubin; increased reticulocytes; increased mean corpuscular hemoglobin count** (>35); decreased MCV; abnormal RBC osmotic lysis test.

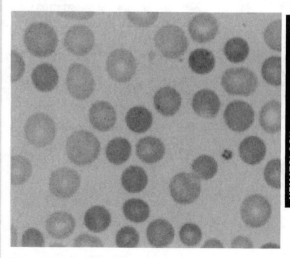

Figure 83-1. Peripheral blood smear.

HEMATOLOGY

case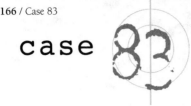

Hereditary Spherocytosis

Differential

Hemolytic Anemia

Biliary Obstruction

Unconjugated Hyperbilirubinemia

Hereditary Elliptocytosis

Discussion

Hereditary spherocytosis is a congenital, **autosomal-dominant** disorder (suggesting that homozygosity is lethal) and is characterized by **hemolytic anemia with spherical RBCs** and splenomegaly. It is caused by a **defect in a RBC membrane spectrin** or associated proteins leading to a defective RBC cytoskeleton with loss of the normal biconcavity and a higher rate of splenic sequestration and hemolysis. If left untreated, it may give rise to pigment **gallstones** and **cholecystitis**.

■ TABLE 83-1 PROTEIN DEFECTS IN HEREDITARY SPHEROCYTOSIS

Spectrin–highest frequency

Ankyrin–binding site for spectrin

Band 3

Protein 4.2 (Pallidin)

Treatment

Folic acid, splenectomy.

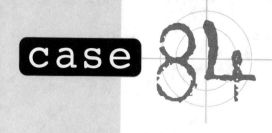

ID/CC   A 1-year-old infant presents at a clinic with **lassitude, poor muscle tone,** and delayed motor development.

HPI   The mother is a known IV drug user and has two older children who are in the custody of the state social services agency. Dietary history indicates no meat but sweet tea and foods low in minerals.

PE   VS: tachycardia; tachypnea. PE: **pallor;** partial alopecia; ulceration of skin at corners of mouth (CHEILOSIS); smooth tongue; **nails break easily** and **are spoon shaped** (KOILONYCHIA).

Labs   PBS: abnormally **small and pale RBCs** (MICROCYTIC, HYPOCHROMIC ANEMIA); RBCs of different sizes (ANISOCYTOSIS) and different shapes (POIKILOCYTOSIS); increased total iron-binding capacity and reduced percentage saturation; **low serum ferritin.**

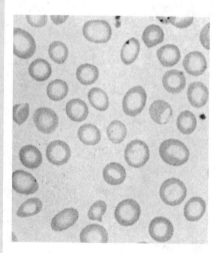

Figure 84-1. Hypochromic, microcytic anemia.

Micro Pathology   Erythroid hyperplasia with **decreased bone marrow iron stores on Prussian blue staining.**

HEMATOLOGY

case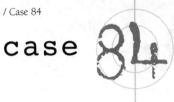

Iron Deficiency Anemia

Differential

Alpha- or Beta-Thalassemia
Hereditary Spherocytosis
Lead Poisoning
Sideroblastic Anemia
Anemia of Chronic Disease

Discussion

Iron-deficiency anemia is the most common cause of **chronic blood loss,** usually gastrointestinal or gynecologic; it is secondary to a deficiency of iron required for normal hemoglobin synthesis. Iron deficiency anemia in an older male and post menopausal female warrants a workup for colon cancer. It should be differentiated from anemia of chronic disease, where ferritin is high and transferrin is low. Iron homeostasis is regulated by absorption into the proximal small intestine.

Treatment

Control cause of iron deficiency; supplemental iron (ferrous sulfate; for children, carbonyl iron).

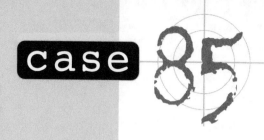

ID/CC   A newborn male in the normal nursery is noted to be **cyanotic;** the pediatrician is called even though the child does not seem to be in respiratory distress.

HPI   That morning he had undergone circumcision (a **benzocaine** ointment was used).

PE   **Cyanotic;** lungs clear and well ventilated; heart sounds rhythmic; no murmurs heard; no cardiopulmonary problems evident.

Labs   CBC/Lytes: normal. Platelets, LFTs, BUN, and creatinine normal. ABGs: **PO$_2$ normal.**

Imaging CXR: normal.

case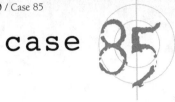

Methemoglobinemia

Differential

Transposition of Great Arteries
Tetralogy of Fallot
Hemoglobinopathies
Pulmonary Embolism
Sepsis

Discussion

Methemoglobin is an oxidized $Fe+3$ (FERRIC) form of hemoglobin (normally $Fe+2$, ferrous) unable to carry oxygen or carbon dioxide. The diminished oxygen-carrying capacity that results produces headache, light-headedness, and dyspnea. The more prominent **acquired methemoglobinemia** involves exposure to **oxidizing drugs** (e.g., dapsone, benzocaine, lidocaine, nitrates, nitrites); **dyes** (anilines) oxidize hemoglobin to its ferric form, as do **enzyme deficiencies** (e.g., cytochrome b5 oxidase, glucose-6-phosphate dehydrogenase). In neonates, **hereditary methemoglobinemia** can involve a transient deficiency of NADH methemoglobin reductase or NADPH flavin reductase, and HbF is more susceptible than HbA to oxidation.

■ **TABLE 85-1 SYMPTOMOLOGY IS PROPORTIONAL TO THE PERCENTAGE OF metHb.**

<10% metHb—No symptoms
10–20% metHb—Skin discoloration (mucous membranes)
20–30% metHb—Headache and dyspnea on exertion
30–50% metHb—Fatigue, tachypnea, palpitations, dizziness
50–70% metHb—Coma, seizures, arrhythmias
>70% metHb—Death

Treatment

Remove precipitating factors; **methylene blue** if severe, although contraindicated in patients with glucose-6-phosphate dehydrogenase deficiency and may lead to severe hemolysis. Ascorbic acid is a coenzyme for reduction.

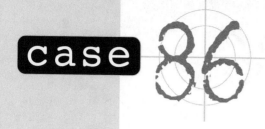

ID/CC A 19-year-old **male** goes to the university clinic complaining of **abdominal and lumbar pain**, which characteristically occurs **when he takes his multivitamin pills** two times a week (iron, infections, and vaccination are precipitating factors); he has also noticed **dark brown urine the morning** after he has the pain (due to hemolysis).

HPI He is a freshman excited about living independently; he likes to drink excessive amounts of beer.

PE Marked **pallor;** lung fields clear to auscultation; heart sounds normal; abdomen soft and nontender with no masses or peritoneal signs; no focal neurologic signs.

Labs CBC: normocytic, normochromic **anemia** with reticulocytosis. **Hemoglobinemia and hemoglobinuria;** absence of CD59 on RBCs by flow cytometry diagnostic; **sucrose hemolysis test positive; acidified serum test positive** (HAM'S TEST); **decreased haptoglobin; elevated LDH; decreased leukocyte alkaline phosphatase.**

Gross Pathology Hemosiderosis of liver, spleen, and kidney.

case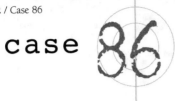

Paroxysmal Nocturnal Hemoglobinuria

Differential

Hemolytic Anemia

Mesenteric Artery Thrombosis or Ischemia

Paroxysmal Cold Hemoglobinuria

Renal Vein Thrombosis

Discussion

Paroxysmal nocturnal hemoglobinuria is an **acquired** defect of the red blood cell membrane, making erythrocytes unusually sensitive to serum complement (also increased binding of C3b), characterized by episodes of hemolysis with hemoglobinuria that occur during sleep by carbon dioxide retention (lowering the pH, thus enhancing complement activity; first voided urine in the morning is red-brown). Patients are also predisposed to developing venous thromboses.

Treatment

Steroids (testosterone analogs or antigonadotropin) to stimulate erthropoiesis, transfusion of RBCs during crises. Oral iron supplementation may be useful but should be used cautiously, as it may precipitate transient hemolysis. Similarly, heparin may accelerate hemolysis, but its use in thrombotic complications appears warranted; use cyclooxygenase inhibitors such as aspirin and ibuprofen.

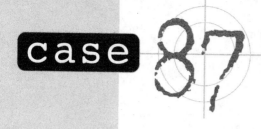

ID/CC A 58-year-old black female complains of **weakness, dizziness,** anorexia, nausea, and occasional vomiting over the past 3 months.

HPI She has also experienced **shortness of breath** as well as **numbness and tingling** in the extremities.

PE Slightly icteric eyes; hepatosplenomegaly; smooth, beefy-red tongue (GLOSSITIS); **"glove and stocking"** distribution of anesthesia; **loss of balance, vibratory, and position sense** in both lower extremities (due to posterior and lateral column involvement; US Folic acid deficiency).

Labs CBC: **macrocytic,** hypochromic anemia (MCV >100); **leukopenia** (4000) with **hypersegmented neutrophils;** thrombocytopenia. Hyperbilirubinemia (2.5 mg/dL; normal 0.1–1.0 mg/dL); **achlorhydria** positive Schilling test.

Micro Pathology **Megaloblastic** and **hypercellular bone marrow** with erythroid hyperplasia; spinal cord shows demyelination and focal vacuolation in white matter with axonal degeneration (Subacute combined degeneration).

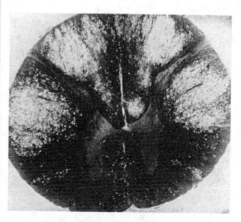

Figure 87-1. Subacute combined degeneration.

HEMATOLOGY

173

case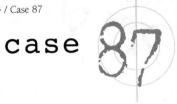

Vitamin B$_{12}$ Deficiency

Differential

HIV-associated Myelopathy

Folate Deficiency

Multiple Sclerosis

Neurosyphilis

Lyme Disease

Discussion

Pernicious anemia is megaloblastic anemia caused by malabsorption of vitamin B$_{12}$ (cobalamin) because of **lack of intrinsic factor (autoimmune antibodies** against gastric intrinsic factor) in gastric juice (intrinsic factor, secreted by parietal cells, is indispensable for vitamin B$_{12}$ absorption). **Antibodies against gastric parietal cells** are almost invariably present in the adult form of the disease. Whereas folate can reverse hematologic abnormalities of B$_{12}$ deficiency, neurological problems such as demyelination is unresolved due to the requirement of adenosylcobalamin, another form of B$_{12}$.

Treatment

Parenteral vitamin B$_{12}$ (cyanocobalamin).

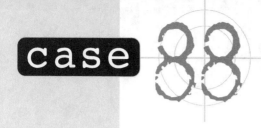

ID/CC A 6-year-old boy is brought to the ER because of **slurred speech, lethargy,** and **severe vomiting.** The patient was "helping" his father in the garage when he saw a bottle and, out of curiosity, drank the sweet liquid.

HPI On arrival at the local pediatric emergency room, the boy started having tonic-clonic **seizures.**

PE VS: tachycardia (HR 108); no fever; **hypotension** (BP 80/40). PE: **hyperventilating** and experiencing **convulsions.**

Labs CBC: leukocytosis (13,000); **metabolic acidosis with elevated osmolar** and **anion gap.** Lytes: hyponatremia; hyperkalemia. BUN and creatinine levels normal. ECG: **premature ventricular beats.**

Imaging CXR: no evidence of bronchoaspiration.

Micro Path Urine sediment with **oxylate crystals.**

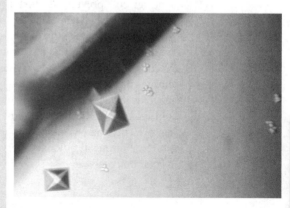

Figure 88-1. Oxylate urine crystals.

case 88

Ethylene Glycol Ingestion

Differential

Alcohol Toxicity

Metabolic Acidosis

Diabetes

Methanol Poisoning

Discussion

Toxicity is due to conversion of these alcohols, themselves relatively nontoxic, to toxic metabolites. Ethylene glycol is the predominant component of antifreeze and may be used by alcoholics as an alcohol substitute. Because of its **sweet taste**, children and pets frequently ingest antifreeze. Its by-products may cause **metabolic acidosis, renal failure (due to intratubular deposition of precipitated oxalate crystals), and death.**

Treatment

Administer ethanol (a substrate with higher affinity; lower Km) to saturate alcohol dehydrogenase (maintain serum level of ~100 mg/dL) and to displace ethylene glycol preventing metabolism to its toxic metabolite glycolate, which is then transformed to glyoxylate, and hence the highly toxic oxalate crystallizing in renal tubules. Administer **pyridoxine** (metabolize glyoxylate to glycine), **folate, and thiamine** (metabolize glycolate to glyoxylate) to attenuate toxic metabolites. Treat convulsions with diazepam and monitor vital signs. **Hemodialysis** can effectively remove ethylene glycol and correct acidosis and electrolyte abnormalities. Rapid intervention is crucial for a good outcome.

case 89

ID/CC A 33-year-old woman presents to a clinic with **marked weakness** (due to hypokalemia).

HPI Two years ago, she underwent an ureterolithotomy for **renoureteral stones.**

PE VS: tachypnea. PE: **generalized muscle weakness;** heart sounds with a few skipped beats (hypokalemia gives rise to severe arrhythmias); diminished intestinal peristalsis; no peritoneal signs.

Labs Lytes: increased urinary potassium excretion (due to insufficient hydrogen ion available, with potassium exchanged for sodium), resulting in **marked hypokalemia** (2.3 mEq/L). ABGs: decreased HCO_3 (due to failure to maintain normal gradient of hydrogen ions in distal renal tubules, with HCO_3 loss); **hyperchloremic metabolic acidosis** (normal anion gap). Normal serum calcium. UA: urine alkaline; hypercalciuria.

Imaging KUB: radiopaque left kidney stones; medullary renal calcification.

Gross Pathology Nephrocalcinosis.

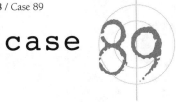

case

Renal Tubular Acidosis

Differential

Nonanion Gap Metabolic Acidosis

Fanconi Syndrome

Drugs (Acetazoliamide, gentamicin)

Vitamin D deficiency

Discussion

Metabolic acidosis is caused by renal tubular defects in transport. **Type I (distal)** involves selective deficiency of tubular H secretion (produces typical hyperchloremic-hypokalemic acidosis with normal anion gap). **Type II (proximal)** involves the inability to reabsorb HCO_3 (also hypokalemic). **Type III** entails the inability to produce NH_3 due to persistently low GFR volumes (normokalemic). **Type IV** is due to primary or drug-induced hypoaldosteronism (hyperkalemic).

■ TABLE 89-1 FEATURES OF RENAL TUBULAR ACIDOSIS

	Distal	Proximal	Type IV
Basic defect	No H^+ in distal tubule	Reduced bicarbonate reabsorption	Decreased K secretion by distal tubule
Urine pH after acid load	>5.4	<5.4	<5.4
Diagnostic test	NH_4CL load	Maximum capacity for HCO_3	Urinary K excretion, renin, aldosterone
Serum K before treatment	Low	Low	High
Serum K after bicarbonate	Normal	Lower	Toward normal
Long-term complications	Renal stones, renal insufficiency	Osteomalacia, growth retardation	None
Associated diseases	Autoimmune	Fanconi syndrome	Diabetes mellitus, interstitial nephritis

Treatment

Alkalinizing agents (sodium bicarbonate, sodium citrate); potassium chloride; diuretics (Furosemide) and vitamin D supplementation (Calcitrol).

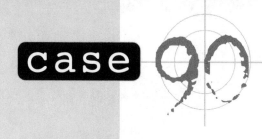

case 90

ID/CC	A 38-year-old electrician is rushed to the emergency room after receiving an accidental high-voltage **electric shock** while fixing a power line.
HPI	On admission, a Foley catheter is inserted, yielding **reddish-brown urine** (due to myoglobin).
PE	VS: tachycardia; BP normal. PE: confusion; disorientation; patient complains of **muscle pain** in right arm, leg, and buttock; hand severely swollen and has an oblique-shaped **burn;** "outlet wound" located in right gluteal region and ankle.
Labs	**Markedly increased serum BUN and creatinine** (due to acute tubular necrosis); urea normal. Lytes: **hyperkalemia.** Hyperphosphatemia; hyperuricemia; hypocalcemia (due to calcium binding to necrotic muscle); **increased serum CK** (due to muscle destruction); **myoglobinuria.**

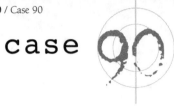

case

Rhabdomyolysis

Differential

Thermal or Electrical Burns

Neuromalignant Syndrome

Cocaine Overdosing

Polymyositis

Myopathies

Discussion

Myoglobinuria and reduced renal perfusion from volume depletion may cause acute tubular damage. Other causes of rhabdomyolysis (**destruction of striated muscle**) that account for 1/7 of acute renal failures include alcohol abuse, crush injuries, seizures, trauma (electrical or thermal burns), drug overdoses, and prolonged unconsciousness in one position. A final outcome is a dysfunction in myocyte calcium homeostasis.

Breakout Point

Causes of Rhabdomyolysis (GIT'EM)
G Genetic (myopathies, enzyme deficiencies)
I   Infection (bacterial, viral)
T Trauma (blunt, burns)
'E Environment/Toxins (alcohol, drugs, carbon monoxide)
M Metabolic (ions)

Treatment

Vigorous **rehydration** (to prevent pigment deposition and acute tubular necrosis) to increase glomerular filtration rate (GFR); urine alkalinization (with IV bicarbonate); osmotic diuretics (mannitol); prevent further muscle damage from compartment syndromes (evaluate need for fasciotomy). Correct electrolyte abnormalities. Hemodialysis may be required in severe cases.

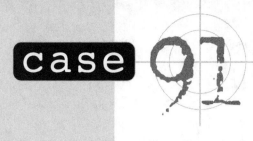

case

ID/CC A 45-year-old male professional soccer player is brought to the emergency room after a complaining of acute **nausea**; he has **vomited** five times, feels very **lightheaded**, and has a severe **headache**.

HPI He went out **drinking** last night to celebrate his team's victory in a soccer tournament he attended last week in Mexico. While in Mexico, he contracted acute amebiasis that is currently being treated with **metronidazole**.

PE VS: marked tachycardia (HR 120); **hypotension** (BP 90/60). PE: anxious, dehydrated, and confused with severe nausea.

Labs CBC/LFTs: normal. Amylase normal. ABG/Lytes: mild hypokalemia and metabolic alkalosis (due to vomiting).

case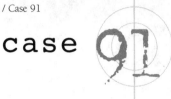

Antabuse Effect (Disulfiram-like Reaction)

Differential

Alcohol Toxicity

Mushroom Toxicity

Gastroenteritis

Discussion

Ethanol is degraded by alcohol dehydrogenase to acetaldehyde, which in turn is degraded to acetic acid by another acetaldehyde dehydrogenase. This **acetaldehyde dehydrogenase is inhibited** by disulfiram, resulting in the **accumulation of acetaldehyde,** which produces nausea, vomiting, headache, and hypotension (ANTABUSE EFFECT). Metronidazole, some cephalosporins, and other drugs have an Antabuse-like effect when consumed concomitantly with alcohol.

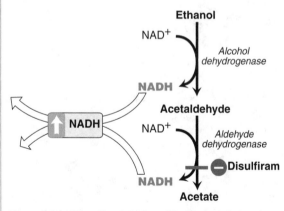

Figure 91-1. Ethanol metabolism. Disulfiram (antabuse) reduces the rate of oxidation of acetaldehyde by competing with the cofactor NAD for binding sites on aldehyde dehydrogenase.

Treatment

Supportive with multiple doses of activated charcoal, IV fluids, antiemetics, discontinuance of alcohol.

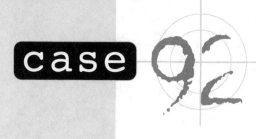

case 92

ID/CC   A 28-year-old male, a chemistry teacher at the local high school, comes to the emergency room complaining of acute **retrosternal and epigastric pain** and frequent **vomiting** of blood-tinged material.

HPI   He admits to bouts of depression and an attempt at **suicide** through the ingestion of several teaspoons of **mercurium bichloride** (corrosive) from his chemistry lab. On arrival at the ER he had a **bloody, diarrheic** bowel movement.

PE   VS: **hypotension**; tachycardia. PE: pallor; skin cold and clammy; tongue whitish; patient is confused, **oliguric, and dyspneic**; moderate abdominal tenderness; **grayish discoloration of buccal mucosa**.

Labs   **Elevated serum creatinine and BUN.** UA: presence of tubular casts. Fractional excretion of sodium markedly increased; serum hemoglobin levels markedly elevated.

Gross Pathology   Acute tubular necrosis; acute irritative colitis with mucosal necrosis with sloughing and hemorrhage.

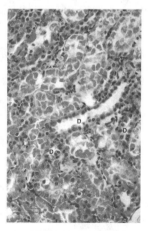

Figure 92-1. There is widespread necrosis of proximal tubular epithelial cells, with sparing of distal and collecting tubules (D) minimal interstitial inflammation.

case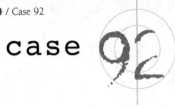

Mercury Toxicity

Differential
Acute Renal Failure
Acute Respiratory Distress Syndrome
Gastroenteritis

Discussion
Mercury, in its multiple forms, is toxic. The patient's outcome depends on the form of the mercury compound and severity of exposure. Organic mercury is the most toxic, and targets the CNS. Acute toxicity by inorganic salts is exemplified by this case and affects corrosive gastroenteritis, acute tubular necrosis. Chronic mercury exposure produces **proteinuria, stomatitis,** and **CNS signs,** mostly in children. These signs include insomnia, irritability, ataxia, nystagmus, and convulsions. Public health concerns target fish consumption (swordfish and tuna) and dental amalgams.

Treatment
Chelation therapy with dimercaprol, succimer (DMSA), and penicillamine; supportive management of acute tubular necrosis; GI decontamination for acute exposure to organic or inorganic mercury. Psychiatric consult for depression.

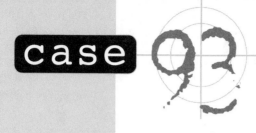

case 93

ID/CC A 4-year-old **male** is brought to the pediatric clinic because of **easy fatigability, difficulty walking, and a waddling gait** of a few months' duration.

HPI The child's mother has noticed that his calves have increased in size (**pseudohypertrophy**).

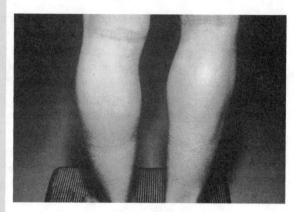

Figure 93-1. Apparent bilateral calf hypertrophy.

PE Child is well developed but shows **proximal muscle weakness** in shoulder and pelvic girdle; difficulty standing and walking; "climbs up on himself" to rise from sitting to standing (GOWERS' SIGN).

Labs CK, LDH, and glucose phosphoisomerase elevated; absent dystrophin expression on immunostain of muscle biopsy.

Gross Pathology Replacement of normal muscle protein with fibrofatty tissue, giving rise to pseudohypertrophy.

Micro Pathology Degeneration and atrophy of muscle fibers with ringed fibers surrounding normal tissue.

case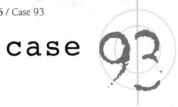

Duchenne Muscular Dystrophy

Differential

Congenital Myopathies

Congenital Muscular Dystrophy

Limb Girdle Muscular Dystrophy

Becker Muscular Dystrophy

Inflammatory Myopathy

Discussion

Duchenne, the most common muscular dystrophy is an **X-linked recessive** disorder characterized by a deficiency in muscle **dystrophin,** a subsarcolemmal cytoskeletal protein engaged in a complex with sarcoglycans and dystroglycans that stabilizes the sarcolemma during contraction and relaxation. Its course is relentlessly progressive, ending in death from cardiac and respiratory muscle involvement.

Treatment

Prognosis is poor, with disability occurring within a few years and death by the early 20s. Treatment is supportive. Refer for genetic counseling.

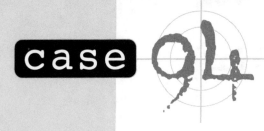

case 94

ID/CC   A 40-year-old male is brought to the ER from a **bar** because of **confusion** after falling from a bar stool.

HPI   The patient's friends say that his diet consists mainly of **alcoholic drinks**. They also state that he tells detailed and **believable stories about his past adventures; subsequently have been found to be untrue** (CONFABULATION). He has **vision abnormalities** and sometimes suffers from double vision (DIPLOPIA). His **short- and long-term memory is severely impaired.**

PE   **Ataxia; oculomotor abnormalities,** including **nystagmus** and **ophthalmoplegia.**

Labs   CBC: macrocytic anemia (most likely secondary to folate deficiency). **Low thiamine (B$_1$) levels.**

Gross Pathology   **Bilateral atrophy of mammillary bodies** and thalamus.

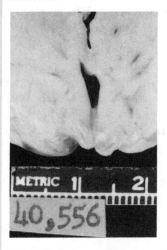

Figure 94-1. A coronal section of brain discloses discoloration and degeneration of the mammillary bodies.

Micro Pathology   Neuronal degeneration in mammillary bodies and thalamus.

187

case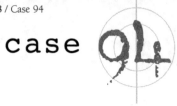

Wernicke–Korsakoff Syndrome

Differential

Alcoholism

Delirium

Dementia Secondary to Head Trauma

Discussion

Wernicke encephalopathy is often **reversible with thiamine (vitamin B$_1$) treatment.** Often associated with alcoholism and chronic liver disease, which attenuates transport and activation of thiamine pyrophosphate to the active thiamine, respectively. A delay in treatment may cause progression to Korsakoff's psychosis with permanent dementia. Patients rarely return to normal. Patients also often have **wet beriberi** (high-output cardiac failure), **dry beriberi** (peripheral neuropathy with impairment of distal motor and sensory function), and cerebral beriberi (motor and cognitive impairment). **Wernicke encephalopathy** consists of a triad of **confusion, ataxia, and ophthalmoplegia.** Korsakoff's psychosis is characterized by **retrograde/anterograde amnesia and confabulation.**

Treatment

Immediate thiamine (B$_1$) administration parenterally can increase attentiveness and orientation. Alcoholics should also receive oral or IV electrolytes, folate, and a multivitamin. Monitor carefully for **delirium tremens** secondary to alcohol withdrawal.

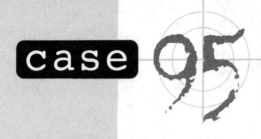

case 95

ID/CC	A 36-year-old female **nonsmoker** visits her family doctor because she has become increasingly **short of breath** (DYSPNEA); her symptoms first appeared only during exercise but now occur even when she is at rest.
HPI	She also complains of frequent URIs and moderate **weight loss.**
PE	**Thin** female with **increased anteroposterior diameter of chest** (BARREL-SHAPED CHEST); decreased breath sounds bilaterally; **hyperresonance** to percussion; retardation of expiratory flow.
Labs	CBC: increased hematocrit. Decreased serum α_1-antitrypsin levels (reference 100–300 mg/dL). PFTs: **FEV$_1$/FVC <75%** (diagnostic of airflow obstruction). ECG: right ventricular hypertrophy.
Imaging	CXR: hyperlucent lung fields; flattening of diaphragm and decreased lung markings at periphery.
Gross Pathology	Destruction of alveolar walls distal to the terminal bronchiole with hyperaeration (EMPHYSEMA); **panacinar type** (COTTON CANDY LUNG); more severe at lung bases.

PULMONARY

case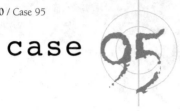

Alpha-1-Antitrypsin Deficiency

Differential

Chronic Obstructive Pulmonary Disease (COPD)

Bronchitis

Emphysema

Discussion

α_1-**antitrypsin** deficiency is one of the most commonly inherited diseases among Caucasians and a leading cause of liver transplantation in children. Pollutants, cigarette smoke, and infections increase PMNs and macrophages in the lung and thus produce a number of proteolytic enzymes. Damage to lung tissue due to these enzymes is controlled by the globulin α_1-**antitrypsin,** which inhibits the neutrophil proteases neutrophil elastase, trypsin, cathepsin G, and collagenase. A deficiency of this enzyme is transmitted as an autosomal-codominant disease and inhibits hepatocytic release causing neutrophil elastase digestion of elastin and collagen in alveolar walls, lung tissue destruction, and **panacinar emphysema.** (Cigarette smoking is associated with the centrilobular type and accelerates the onset of symptoms.) Patients may also develop **liver damage** due to excess buildup of this protein in the liver.

Treatment

Standard treatment for COPD patients. Replacement therapy with α_1-protease inhibitor. Lung transplantation, preferably prior to development of pulmonary hypertension.

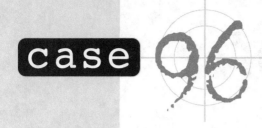

case 96

ID/CC A 36-year-old divorcee living in rural Maine is brought by ambulance to the ER with her two children, who were **all found unconscious in her home** by military personnel.

HPI A recent "El Niño" produced bad weather that resulted in a power failure; as a result, she had been using charcoal and a **wooden stove inside her house** for heating purposes.

PE **Skin bright red** (CHERRY-RED CYANOSIS); pulse arrhythmic; patient regains consciousness soon after administration of 100% oxygen but remains drowsy, **disoriented,** and nauseous and complains of a severe **headache** (due to cerebral edema); **hyperreflexia** noted as well as positive Romberg's test. VS: **tachycardia** (HR 90); hypertension (BP 140/90) (no tachypnea).

Labs **Increased carboxyhemoglobin** (>25%). ABGs: metabolic acidosis.

Imaging CT/MR: bilateral globus pallidus lesions.

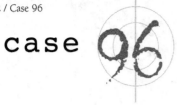

case 96

Carbon Monoxide Poisoning

Differential

Anemia

Inhalation Injury

Migraine Headache

Stroke

Discussion

As the leading cause of death by poisoning, sources of CO are: automobile exhaust, pipes, and smoke inhalation from fires. Carbon monoxide has a much greater affinity for hemoglobin than oxygen (250 times more). If the patient is pregnant, damage to the fetus is devastating (HbF has greater affinity to CO than HbA). CO binds HbA 250 times more avidly than O_2 and causes increased O_2 binding at the other 3 oxygen binding sites, causing a leftward shift in the oxyhemoglobin dissociation curve and decreasing O_2 availability to already hypoxic tissues. Long-term side effects such as memory problems, lack of coordination, and even convulsions are common after intoxication.

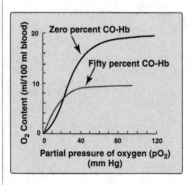

Figure 96-1. Effect of carbon monoxide on oxygen affinity to hemoglobin.

Treatment

One hundred percent **oxygen** until patient asymptomatic, assisted ventilation if necessary. Hyperbaric oxygen chamber.

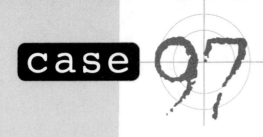

case 97

ID/CC	A **premature** (32-week-old) white male infant is brought to the pediatric intensive care unit after a **cesarean** delivery.
HPI	His mother, a diabetic, had third-trimester **bleeding** and contractions that did not stop with rest and conservative treatment.
PE	VS: tachypnea. PE: child weighs 3.8 lb; **cyanosis; dyspnea;** uses accessory muscles of respiration; **nasal flaring.**
Labs	ABGs: hypoxemia; hypercapnia. Decreased lecithin/sphingomyelin (L/S) ratio (normally >2; 1.5–2.0 in 40% of newborns with respiratory distress).
Imaging	CXR: bilateral **reticular pulmonary infiltrates,** air bronchograms, and atelectasis.

PULMONARY

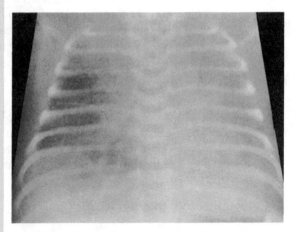

Figure 97-1. The chest radiograph shows hypoaeration, diffusely opaque lung fields, air bronchograms, and loss of normal vascular shadows.

Gross Pathology	Generalized atelectasis in purple-colored lung; eosinophilic fibrinous hyaline membrane formation.

193

case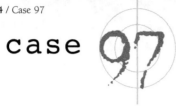

Hyaline Membrane Disease

Differential

Aspiration Syndromes

Pneumonia

Pneumothorax

Discussion

Also known as **respiratory distress syndrome (RDS)**; it is the most common cause of death in premature infants. The severity of the disease is inversely proportional to the gestational age of the infant. It is due to a **deficiency of surfactant**, a complex lipoprotein produced by type II pneumocyte cells containing the phospholipid lecithin (dipalmitoyl phosphatidylcholine) along with other phospholipid and lipoprotein components causing spreading of lecithin as a monolayer, lowering the surface tension of the alveolar air/fluid interface. Fetal lung maturity may be measured by the L/S ratio. RDS might be prevented by giving **betamethasone** to pregnant women, since type II pneumocyte cell differentiation is **steroid**-dependent. Complications include: patent ductus arteriosus, pulmonary air leaks, and bronchopulmonary dysplasia.

Treatment

Ventilatory support, fluid, acid-base and electrolyte balance, antibiotics; administration of surfactant (most infants with RDS require 2 doses); steroids before birth to speed lung maturity.

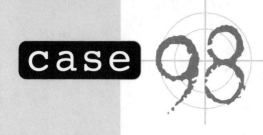

ID/CC   A 23-year-old female college student is brought to the emergency room because of **numbness** of her face and feet together with a **sensation of suffocation** and **stiff twisting of the hands** (CARPOPEDAL SPASM); these symptoms arose following an argument with her boyfriend.

HPI   A friend reports that the patient has a **history of anxiety-induced colitis, gastritis, and migraine.**

PE   VS: **marked tachypnea** (RR 40); tachycardia (HR 90); hypertension (BP 140/90). PE: patient **apprehensive** and anxious; physical exam otherwise normal.

Labs   ABGs: **low Pco$_2$; respiratory alkalosis** (cause of tetany); **low bicarbonate** (to compensate for primary lowering of Pco$_2$).

Imaging   CXR: normal

PULMONARY

case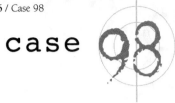

Hyperventilation

Differential

Acute Respiratory Distress Syndrome
Cardiomyopathy
Pulmonary Embolism

Discussion

Anxiety hyperventilation is a common occurrence in ERs, and can comprise up to 10% of internal medicine cases with many false diagnoses. The anxiety state produces an increase in the frequency of respirations (HYPERVENTILATION), where ventilation exceeds metabolic demands causing a **lowering of P_{CO_2}**; the resulting respiratory alkalosis produces an unstable depolarization of the distal segments of motor nerves with symptomatic tetany. Alkalosis also sets in motion a compensatory decrease in bicarbonate level to maintain pH as close to normal as possible. There is a left shift of the HbO2 dissociation curve.

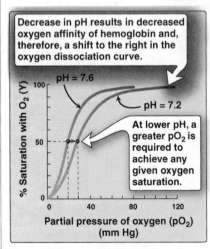

Figure 98-1. Alkalosis by hyperventilation yields a decrease in bicarbonate level to maintain pH with a left shift of the HbO2 dissociation curve.

Treatment

Have patient **breathe in and out of a bag** or give 5% CO_2 mixture. Benzodiazepines (Alprazolam) to reduce stress.

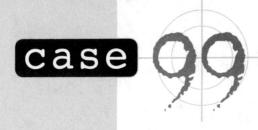
ID/CC A 25-year-old male visits a fertility clinic as part of an **evaluation of infertility** that he is undergoing with his wife.

HPI His medical history discloses frequent **sinus infec-tions** (SINUSITIS), chronic cough with sputum forma-tion, and recurrent ear infections.

PE VS: normal. PE: apical impulse felt on fifth **right intercostal space;** all auscultatory foci reversed (DEX-TROCARDIA); liver on left side and spleen on right (SITUS INVERSUS).

Labs CBC/Lytes: normal. Semen analysis shows **immotile spermatozoa.**

Imaging CXR: hyperinflation, bronchiectasis, and dextro-cardia. KUB: situs inversus. CT: sinuses: opacified sinuses; mucosal thickening.

PULMONARY

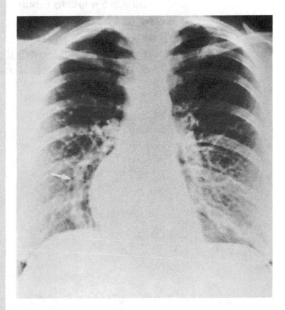

Figure 99-1. Situs inversus.

197

case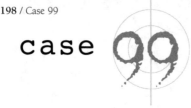

Kartagener Syndrome

Differential

Alpha-1-antitrypsin deficiency

Cystic Fibrosis

Allergic Bronchopulmonary Aspergillosis

Pulmonary Sequestration

Chronic Aspiration

Discussion

Kartagener syndrome (also called immotile cilia syndrome or primary ciliary dyskinesia) is an **autosomal-recessive** disorder characterized by a reduction in the number of **dynein** (ATPASE) arms from the microtubules of axonemes in the cilia of the sinuses and bronchi, rendering them immotile. Sperm are also immotile (due to flagellar lack of dynein). The lack of mucus-clearing action causes frequent infections.

Breakout Point

Clinical Symptoms (BIAS)
B Bronchiectasis
I Immobility of cilia
A Abnormal sinusitis (frontal sinuses)
S Situs inversus (transposition) of viscera

Treatment

Antibiotics directed against pathogens identified in sputum; mucolytics to reduce viscosity of mucous secretions; IVF for fertility issues.

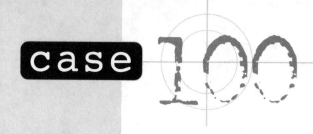
ID/CC A 52-year-old obese white male comes to his family doctor complaining of severe pain in the **first metatarsophalangeal (MTP) joint** (PODAGRA) that began at **night** after an episode of binge **eating** and **drinking.**

HPI He admits to being an avid **meat** eater and drinks **red wine** every night. His history is significant for removal of **kidney stones** (uric acid stones).

PE VS: **fever** (38.2°C). PE: **right MTP joint** red, hot, and swollen; painful to active and passive motion; **tophaceous** deposits in left ear and olecranon bursitis.

Labs **Elevated serum uric acid.** UA: urate crystals. **Increased ESR.** CBC: leukocytosis with neutrophilia.

Imaging XR: punched-out erosions in right big toe at MTP joint, producing **"overhanging"** spicules.

Gross Pathology Tophi are white, soft, nodular masses of urate deposits with calcifications seen mainly in synovial membranes, tendon sheaths, and ear cartilages.

Micro Pathology Tophi and synovial fluid aspiration show characteristic negatively **birefringent, needle-shaped crystals** of uric acid salts; giant cell formation with neutrophilic infiltration.

RHEUMATOLOGY

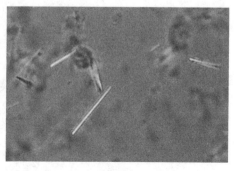

Figure 100-1. Negatively birefringent, long, needle-shaped crystals of uric acid.

199

case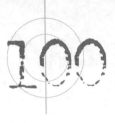

Gout

Differential	Rheumatoid Arthritis
	Uric Acid Nephropathy
	Pseudogout
	Septic Arthritis
	Sarcoidosis
Discussion	Gout is a disorder of purine metabolism with a resulting increase in serum uric acid level and deposits in several tissues; 10% to 20% of cases may develop nephrolithiasis. In late stages, urate deposits in the kidney may lead to chronic pyelonephritis, arteriolar sclerosis, hypertension, and renal failure.
Treatment	NSAIDs (indomethacin) for acute symptoms, Colchicine for initial onset 12–24 hours; long-term treatment with a xanthine oxidase inhibitor (Allopurinol) and/or a uricosuric agent (Probenecid).

questions

1. A three year old boy who recently immigrated with his parents from a war torn area of Yugoslavia comes to the emergency room of the city hospital in the early afternoon, complaining of acute abdominal pain, malaise and an abscess on his arm. Examination by the ER physician notes very dark urine, icteric sclerae. A stool sample contains undigested beans and upon inquiry, they are revealed to be fava beans. Laboratory results indicate hemoglobin 6.5 g/dL, hematocrit low with reticulocytes at 7%, and direct bilirubin is elevated. Urinalysis is positive for blood. The disorder that fits this patient's profile is:

   A. Alkaptonuria
   B. Glucose 6-phosphate dehydrogenase deficiency
   C. Paroxysmal nocturnal hemoglobinuria
   D. Sickle cell anemia
   E. Spherocytosis (hereditary)

2. A seven-year-old male is referred to a genetic evaluation clinic by his pediatrician because of mental retardation (decreasing IQ with age) and behavioral problems. The parents, considering another child, wished an evaluation. Upon physical examination, the child has a midsystolic click in the mitral area and large jaw and ears. What is the most likely genetic mutation present in this patient?

   A. Frameshift mutation
   B. Missense mutation
   C. Nonsense mutation
   D. Silent mutation
   E. Trinucleotide repeat expansion

3. An 11-year-old female presents to the internal medicine clinic with her father who is a popular macrobiotic diet expert. He reports that his daughter has a recent history of severe headache, diplopia, and bone pain. A physical examination indicates moderate acne and papilledema with a fundoscopic examination. What vitamin derangement is most likely being exhibited in this patient?

   A. Vitamin A deficiency
   B Vitamin A toxicity
   C. Vitamin C deficiency
   D. Vitamin C toxicity
   E. Vitamin B_3 deficiency

4. A 53-year-old female passes out at work and is brought to the emergency department at the local hospital. Her blood sugar is 21 mg/dl (normal >70). She is also tested for C-peptide, which is much higher than normal. She has never been tested for diabetes before, though there is a family history of Type 1. What is a possible cause of this woman's state?

   A. Anorexia
   B. High protein diet
   C. Diabetic ketoacidosis
   D. Exogenous administration of insulin
   E. Insulin secreting islet cell tumor

5. A 41-year-old man was taken by ambulance after succumbing to pain during a leisurely bicycle ride through the park. He presents to the emergency room complaining of chest discomfort with exertion. Both electrocardiogram and blood labs confirm a cardiac ischemic event. His cholesterol level is 475. He appears healthy for his age but has clusters of small yellow surface nodules around his eyes. He states that both his father and paternal grandmother died of "heart attacks" in their mid-50s. His presentation is most likely a result from a defect in:

   A. Cholesterol synthesis
   B. Apoprotein C
   C. HMG-CoA reductase
   D. LDL receptor
   E. Lipoprotein lipase

6. A 36-year-old pregnant woman, at 36 weeks' gestation, without prenatal care, presents to obstetrics ward at the public hospital. The infant is delivered vaginally, after a relatively short labor without complications. Evaluation of the infant reveals severe cardiomegaly and normal blood sugar levels. Accumulation of glycogen in cytosolic vacuoles is noted. Which enzyme is most likely deficient?

   A. Glucose-6-phosphatase
   B. Alpha-1,4 glucosidase
   C. Debranching enzyme
   D. Glycogen phosphorylase
   E. Alpha galactosidase A

7. A 17-year-old female about to enter college is required to have a physical examination. She goes to a gynecology clinic and expresses little concern that she has never had a menstrual period. Physical exam reveals a marked absence of axillary and pubic hair. The patient has breast tissue present bilaterally. Pelvic exam reveals the vagina ending in a blind pouch. Bimanual exam reveals absence of cervix, uterus, and ovaries. What is the most likely karyotype of this patient?

A. 45, XO
B. 46, XX (5 alpha reductase deficiency)
C. 46, XX (17 alpha hydroxylase deficiency)
D. 46, XY
E. 47, XXY

8. A 32-year-old black steakhouse owner eats at her restaurant, drinks a few beers at mealtime and before bed, and notices a dull ache in her hip. The pain increased to an extent where she went to the emergency department and was admitted. On admission, her temperature was 101°F, and there was a slightly elevated pulse rate. She thought she had broken her toe on several occasions, but "it healed fast." Physical examination was unremarkable. X-ray examination of the abdomen and pelvis yielded no abnormalities. Urinalysis revealed cloudy, acidic urine, with protein in the urine. After centrifugation, the sediment revealed fine crystalline material. She is diagnosed with gout, a disease in which uric acid crystal deposits in joints cause severe pain. Xanthine oxidase converts hypoxanthine to uric acid. To decrease the serum uric acid level, allopurinol is prescribed. The action of allopurinol is in:

A. Binding to the active site of hypoxanthine-guanine phosphoribosyl transferase.
B. Competing directly with xanthine oxidase since they have a similar structure.
C. Acting upon xanthine oxidase directly and inactivates it.
D. Binding to hypoxanthine and prevents it from binding to xanthine oxidase.
E. Binding to a site on xanthine oxidase that is distinct from the active site.

9. A 49-year-old patient presents to his physician with the complaints of weight loss and fatigue. He has delayed seeing the doctor for months, in denial of what might be occurring to his health. A work-up in childhood was remarkable for a deficiency in the enzyme tyrosinase. Which cancer has most likely transpired and is responsible for his symptomology?

A. Squamous cell carcinoma
B. Fanconi anemia
C. Carcinoid tumors
D. Insulinoma
E. Adenocarcinoma of the colon

10. A 41-year-old woman has given birth to a baby boy who has growth retardation, microcephaly, and a cardiac murmur. The woman has had three previous late-term miscarriages and has a 5-year-old girl who is suffering from mental retardation. The maternal condition consistent with this history is:

A. Type 1 diabetes mellitus
B. Type 2 adult onset diabetes
C. Fragile X syndrome
D. Homocystinuria
E. Phenylketonuria

11. A 22-year-old is rushed to the emergency department with nonspecific seizures. Laboratory tests indicated low serum sodium, normal potassium, inappropriately concentrated urine (urinary sodium 60 meq/L), and inhibition of rennin-angiotensin-aldosterone system. The most likely explanation of these findings indicates that the patient has:

A. Syndrome of inappropriate secretion of antidiuretic hormone
B. Congestive heart failure
C. Hyponatremia
D. Renal failure—acute
E. Addison disease

12. A 25-year-old rural resident sprayed "a bit" of parathion on her soybean crops. She became nauseated, vomited, had diarrhea, cramps, and dizziness with blurred vision. As time progressed she had difficulty talking, became weak, sweated profusely, and had miosis (small pupils). BP 170/115, HR 120 beats/min. Upon workup the patient became agitated, salivated profusely, and was lacrimating (tearing). In an hour severe abdominal cramps and urinary and fecal incontinence ensued. Blood tests indicated cholinesterase was 1/10th normal. Administration of pralidoxime is initiated in what manner?

A. A slow administration that will displace the inhibitor of the enzyme.

B. A quick administration to displace the inhibitor and restore enzyme function before denaturation.

C. A race to reactivate cholinesterase before "aging" occurs and it is altered permanently by covalent bond.

D. A slow administration of a chemical mimicking the structure of the inhibitor that does not bind at the active site.

E. A quick administration of a chemical mimicking the structure of the inhibitor that does not bind at the active site to restore enzyme function before denaturation.

13. An 8-week-old, breast fed, white infant girl is brought to the family medicine clinic with diarrhea, extensive bruising, and GI bleeding. Labs indicate that there are extended prothrombin and partial thromboplastin times, normal platelet count and fibrinogen level, and severe anemia (Hb 19). The cause of the bleeding is most likely due to:

A. Factor V deficiency

B. Factor VIII deficiency

C. Factor XII deficiency

D. Vitamin K deficiency

E. Hepatic disease

14. A 36-year-old male visits his internist with headaches and diaphoresis brought on by stress or exercise. He is found to have a severe hypertension and an abdominal CT indicates a 4-cm mass consistent with a pheochromocytoma. The diagnosis is confirmed with a 24-hour urine collection measuring several catecholamines. The initial treatment regimen commences with:

A. A dopamine receptor blocker

B. An alpha adrenergic receptor blocker

C. A beta adrenergic receptor blocker

D. An angiotensin converting enzyme inhibitor

E. A selective serotonin reuptake inhibitor

15. An 11-month-old, very pale boy is being evaluated for anemia. His nourishment is derived from goat milk exclusively for the last six months. Baby food and cereals have not been introduced in the diet. Laboratory findings include: hemoglobin of 5.7 g/dL, and white blood cell count and platelets were decreased. The differential count with ovalocytic erythrocytes was: 31% neutrophils with hypersegmentation, 67% lymphocytes, and 2% monocytes. The most likely cause of this anemia is:

A. Fanconi anemia
B. Vitamin B_{12} deficiency
C. Vitamin E deficiency
D. Folate deficiency
E. Iron deficiency

16. A 20-year-old white male receives an internal medicine consult for a URI with accompanying jaundice occurring when minor infections ensue. The family history, devoid of consanguinity, indicates that the patient's father had mild cases of unconjugated hyperbilrubinemia and a paternal grandmother who had bouts of fatigue accompanied by mild sclaeral icterus. Based on the family history, the inheritance pattern of this hyperbilirubinemia is most likely:

A. Mitochondrial
B. Autosomal dominant
C. Autosomal recessive
D. X-linked dominant
E. X-linked recessive

17. A 31-year-old female fractured her pelvis during gymnastics practice and is recuperating in a cast immobilized at home. She complains of progressive constipation, polyuria, and fatigue. Her significant other reports that she irregularly takes a multivitamin supplement and is irritable compared to her "old self." The cause of her complaints are most likely:

A. Hyperkalemia
B. Hypercalcemia
C. Hypocalcemia
D. Hypermagnesemia
E. Hypomagnesemia

18. A 4-week-old baby who has been breast fed exclusively is admitted to the pediatric intensive care unit because of lethargy, hypotonia, inability to suck for prolonged time, and jaundice. Postpartum the baby was not jaundiced. Labs indicate that bilirubin is elevated with 30% of total is conjugated. Sepsis caused by E. coli is present. Jaundice in this infant is most consistent with the diagnosis of:

A. Cystic fibrosis
B. Galactosemia
C. Homocystinuria
D. Intolerance to fructose
E. Maple syrup urine disease

19. A 2-year-old child is brought to the pediatrics clinic for evaluation of failure to thrive, fatigue, and sweating profusely. Family history indicates the parents are consanguineous. Physical examination reveals hepatomegaly, protuberant abdomen, and purpuric patches on his skin. Laboratory results indicate lactic acidosis, hyperuricemia, hypoglycemia, and hyperlipidemia. Management of this disease over the course of a lifetime involves administration of:

    A. Medium chain triglycerides orally
    B. L-carnitine orally
    C. Protein orally
    D. 5% dextrose intravenously
    E. Cornstarch orally

20. An 8-month-old male infant of Ashkenazi Jewish parents is brought to clinic due to failure to thrive. Parents also complain of complete lack of social activity, failure to reach for objects, and decreased muscle tone. An ophthalmologic examination yields cherry red spots on the macula. These findings of a metabolic defect are most consistent with:

    A. Hunter syndrome
    B. Hurler syndrome
    C. Niemann-Pick disease
    D. Metachromatic leukodystrophy
    E. Tay-Sachs disease

answers

1-B

A. Alkaptonuria [Incorrect] is an inborn error of metabolism where urine becomes black because of a deficiency of the hepatic enzyme homogentisate 1,2-dioxygenase, which yields an accumulation of homogentisic acid that when oxidizes becomes black. There is no report of this disorder and it should be identified by this age.

B. Glucose 6-phosphate dehydrogenase deficiency [Correct] maintains glutathione in its reduced form crucial for erythrocytes where proteins need to be maintained oxidative stress-free. This patient has an infection to start with and the ingestion of fava beans sensitizes the Mediterranean variant and exacerbates hemolysis.

C. Paroxysmal nocturnal hemoglobinuria [Incorrect] usually occurs in the night and not coincident with the time of the ER visit or changes in pallor. Furthermore, blood labs did not come back positive for hemolysis that caused elevations in LDH or decreased leukocytic alkaline phosphatase.

D. Sickle cell anemia [Incorrect] is not considered since the origin of the boy is in Eastern Europe and there is no indication from blood labs of sickling.

E. Spherocytosis (hereditary) [Incorrect] has a main feature of splenomegaly that is not present in this patient.

2-E

A. Frameshift mutation [Incorrect] caused by the addition or deletion of a base pair, which changes the reading frame. The resultant protein is usually nonfunctional and may be truncated due to a premature stop codon.

B. Missense mutation [Incorrect]. This in-frame mutation replaces a base for the "normal" base resulting in a coding mutation. The classic example is sickle cell anemia caused by a point mutation in which glutamic acid is replaced with valine. The result is an unstable hemoglobin molecule.

C. Nonsense mutation [Incorrect] causes an insertion of a stop codon in the reading frame. The resultant protein is usually truncated and nonfunctional.

D. Silent mutation [Incorrect] changes the codon but still specifies the same amino acid since there is degeneracy in the genetic code, usually occurs in the third "wobble" base of the triplet. There is no adverse reaction from this type of mutation.

E. Trinucleotide repeat expansion [Correct] as in Fragile X syndrome where triplet codons are amplified in tandem. In Fragile X syndrome and myotonic dystrophy this expansion occurs in the noncoding region whereas in Huntington disease this expansion causes glutamine residues within the protein. Severity of these disorders is usually proportional to the number of repeats.

3-B

A. Vitamin A deficiency [Incorrect]. Vitamin A deficiency presents with decreased visual acuity, especially night vision. Physical exam often shows dry eyes, xerophthalmia.

B. Vitamin A toxicity [Correct]. The symptoms are consistent with pseudotumor cerebri. There can be heptomegaly, cirrhosis, and scaly skin. As a fat soluble retinoid this vitamin is stored and not excreted from the body.

C. Vitamin B$_3$ [Incorrect] deficiency, pellagra, has the triad of dementia, dermatitis, and diarrhea as the most common symptoms. This is most common in alcoholics and may be associated with other B vitamin deficiencies.

D. Vitamin C deficiency [Incorrect] presents in patients as scurvy. This leads to the above connective tissue abnormalities. Treatment is oral ascorbic acid (vitamin C).

E. Vitamin C toxicity [Incorrect] is fairly rare as this water soluble vitamin is fairly well tolerated. Overdosing can cause hemolytic crises with G6PD deficiency and diarrhea.

4-E

A. Anorexia [Incorrect] would not cause her blood glucose to drop that precipitously and would not account for elevated C-peptide.

B. A high protein diet [Incorrect] connotes not eating high carbohydrates, which is not a large enough stimulus to result in a high insulin or corresponding C-peptide level.

C. Diabetic ketoacidosis [Incorrect] is not indicated because there is no vomiting or diarrhea and no fruity breath based upon ketone bodies.

D. Exogenous administration of insulin [Incorrect] is contraindicated since if she was self-administering pharmaceutical insulin it would not include C-peptide; therefore her serum C-peptide level would not be elevated.

E. Insulin secreting islet cell tumor or insulinoma [Correct] would be indicated since the pancreas synthesizes proinsulin, which is cleaved in the Golgi apparatus to insulin and C-peptide.

5-D

A. A defect in cholesterol synthesis [Incorrect] would result in hypocholesterolemia.

B. HMG-CoA reductase deficiency [Incorrect] (the same phenotype as if the patient was taking statins) would decrease cholesterol synthesis.

C. Apolipoprotein C [Incorrect] (the activator of lipoprotein lipase) deficiency would result in xanthomas but is inherited recessively in its familial form.

D. A defect in LDL receptor [Correct] implying familial hypercholesterolemia would result in the xanthomas around his eyes and coronary artery disease and fits the autosomal dominant familial inheritance pattern.

E. Lipoprotein lipase deficiency [Incorrect] would result in xanthomas but is inherited recessively in its familial form.

6-B

A. Glucose-6-phosphatase. [Incorrect] Von Gierke disease (type I glycogen storage disease) is associated with severe hypoglycemia, elevated lactic acid, and high levels of uric acid. The liver is enlarged and fatty. Glycogen in these patients appears normal.

B. Alpha-glucosidase. [Correct] Pompe disease (type II glycogen storage disease) is associated with cardiomegaly and early death. Glycogen accumulates in cytosolic vacuoles throughout the body, including heart, liver, and muscle. Blood sugar remains normal. Glycogen in these patients appears normal.

C. Debranching enzyme. [Incorrect] Cori disease (type III glycogen storage disease) presents with hypoglycemic seizures early in life, with eventual hepatic disease and progressive muscle weakness. Dextrin accumulates in the cytosol. Since glycogen branches with (1,6) sugar linkages cannot be metabolized, glycogen retains short branches.

D. Glycogen phosphorylase. [Incorrect] McArdle syndrome (type V glycogen storage disease) is a glycogen phosphorylase deficiency limited to skeletal muscle. Affected patients develop weakness and cramping after exercise, without lactate elevation. Myoglobulinuria is possible in adults. No mental retardation is associated. Glycogen in these patients appears normal.

E. Alpha galactosidase A. [Incorrect] Deficiency of this enzyme (Fabry disease) is involved in glycosphingolipid metabolism with ceramide trihexoses accumulating in the brain. As a lysosomal storage disease, this is irrelevant to glycogen metabolism.

7-D

A. 45, XO. [Incorrect] Patients with 45, XO karyotype have Turner's syndrome. These patients have short stature, webbing of the neck, a broad chest with wide spaced nipples, and possible heart defects (coarctation of the aorta, valvular defects).

B. 46, XX. [Incorrect] The patient with 5-alpha-reductase deficiency has ambiguous external genitalia, hyperkalemia, and hyponatremia due to a decrease in cortisol with a consequent increase in ACTH.

C. 46, XX. [Incorrect] The patient with 17-alpha-hydroxylase deficiency has impaired sex steroid and cortisol biosynthesis. Females fail to develop secondary sexual characteristics and have neither pubic hair, axillary hair, nor breast development, but present with extreme hypertension (unlike this case).

D. 46, XY. [Correct] The patient above has androgen insensitivity syndrome, also known as testicular feminization syndrome. These patients have a 46, XY karyotype and also have testicles, which may be present in the inguinal canal area or intrabdominally. Testes should be removed because they have a high incidence of developing cancer.

E. 47, XXY. [Incorrect] Klinefelter's syndrome patients with 47, XXY have a male phenotype. They typically have a very tall, eunuchoid body habitus with small testes. They may also have breast enlargement and mild mental retardation. This is the most common type of male hypogonadism.

8-C

A. Hypoxanthine-guanine phosphoribosyl transferase (HGPRT) [Incorrect], while involved in the purine salvage pathway, is associated with Lesch-Nyhan syndrome and is not directly related to the etiology of hypouricemia.

B. Allopurinol, [Incorrect] a small molecule drug, does not have a similar structure to enzyme xanthine oxidase, which is a large enzyme–protein complexed with molybdenum.

C. Allopurinol [Correct] does interact directly to inhibit the enzyme xanthine oxidase, by virtue of being a competitive inhibitor with the substrate hypoxanthine, meaning the molecular structures are similar. Allopurinol inhibits the conversion of hypoxanthine to uric acid which precipitates causing the symptomology of gout.

D. Allopurinol [Incorrect] does not directly bind to hypoxanthine but is an analogue that competes for binding to the enzyme at the active site.

E. Allopurinol [Incorrect] does not bind to any site distinct from the active site cleft of the enzyme. If so, then the mode of inhibition would be noncompetitive.

9-A

A. Squamous cell carcinoma (basal cell carcinoma, melanoma) [Correct] are skin cancers that patients with albinism are prone to contract due to a tyrosinase deficiency precluding melanin formation. Patients with albinism are vulnerable to developing skin cancer; melanomas are nonpigmented rather than black since there is no melanin formation.

B. Fanconi anemia [Incorrect] is a congenital disorder of one of 11 genes characterized by constitutional aplastic anemia due to defective DNA repair that can lead to other solid tumors.

C. Carcinoid tumors [Incorrect] arise from the GI system or bronchi and involve hypersecretion of serotonin.

D. Insulinoma [Incorrect] is the most common pancreatic islet cell endocrine tumor and is usually benign.

E. Adenocarcinoma of the colon [Incorrect] is not involved with a higher incidence in patients with Type I albinism.

10-E

A. Though women with Type 1 diabetes [Incorrect] can give birth to infants with neural tube defects and congenital heart disease, mental retardation is not a risk.

B. Type 2 diabetics [Incorrect] do not exhibit risks associated with the case above, and mental retardation is not indicated.

C. Fragile X syndrome [Incorrect] is an X-linked disorder that has mental retardation as a feature in both sex offspring, but males are more likely to have macrocephaly. There is no predilection for miscarriage during pregnancy.

D. In homocystinuria [Incorrect] there is mental retardation in offspring, but there is no indication that the accompanying diminished visual acuity and marfanoid characteristics (tall, thin with elongated limbs) are present.

E. If maternal levels of phenylalanine are high [Correct], growth and mental retardation, microcephaly, and congenital heart defects can occur even if the fetus does not exhibit PKU. Among children of women with untreated PKU, the incidence of mental retardation can be as high as 90%.

11-A

A. In the syndrome of inappropriate secretion of antidiuretic hormone (SIADH) [Correct] the hallmark involves the inappropriate concentration of urine in the absence of mitigating circumstances such as renal or liver failure, hypothyroidism, or adrenal disorders. There is hyponatremia, normokalemia, and inappropriately concentrated urine (urinary Na >20 meq/L) The problem is water retention, not sodium wasting, therefore water restriction.

B. Congestive heart failure [Incorrect] can be ruled out since there is usually accompanying edema and hypervolemia.

C. In generic hyponatremia [Incorrect] routine labs are present other than low sodium and is usually iatrogenic in nature.

D. In acute renal failure [Incorrect] accompanied by oliguria, free water intake exceeds urine volume to cause hyponatremia. There should be accompanying indicators of compromised renal failure such as elevated creatinine.

E. Addison disease [Incorrect] results in adrenal insufficiency through autoimmune destruction of the adrenal cortex. There is no evidence of gonadal failure, vomiting, vitiligo, and there is usually hyperkalemia—not present in this case.

12-C

Organophosphate (pesticide/herbicide) intoxication is caused by the irreversible inhibition of acetylcholinesterase as evidenced by the worsening of symptoms as time progresses. The antidote reactivates the enzyme and removes the phosphoryl group. A hallmark of irreversible inhibitors is the time dependency to treat to reactivate the enzyme before "aging" occurs and it is permanently altered by a covalent bond with the phosphoryl group.

A. A slow administration is not optimal since time is of the essence [Incorrect].

B. A quick administration to displace the inhibitor implies that there is mimicry with the inhibitor that is not the case here [Incorrect].

C. Immediate reactivation is required prior to "aging" and formation of a covalent bond with the inhibitor's phosphoryl group [Correct].

D. A slow administration is not optimal since formation of a covalent bond with the inhibitor is the goal [Incorrect].

E. This is not competitive inhibition, so speed of administration is not an issue [Incorrect].

13-D

A. Factor V [Incorrect] proaccelerin is not vitamin K dependent, so is not deficient.

B. Factor VIII, [Incorrect] the factor whose absence is the cause of hemophilia A, is neither vitamin K dependent nor deficient.

C. Factor XII, [Incorrect] or Hageman factor, is also not vitamin K dependent and is not deficient.

D. Vitamin K deficiency [Correct] is indicated in newborn hemorrhagic disorders, by limited synthesis in the immature liver. In a breast-fed newborn, antibodies contribute delaying bacterial colonization, another source of vitamin K. Through gamma carboxylation, vitamin K is required for coagulation factors II, VII, IX, X.

E. Hepatic disease [Incorrect] would also cause delayed prothrombin and partial thromboplastin times and vitamin K dependent processes, BUT fibrinogen and Factor V are normal.

14-B

Pheochromocytomas are tumors of the adrenal medulla that primarily secrete epinephrine or norepinephrine and to a lesser extent, dopamine. Often there is increased urinary excretion of catecholamines and the symptoms above. Hypertension is treated first prior to tumor resection.

A. An increase of dopamine [Incorrect] is usually indicated with neuroblastomas, and these receptor blockers are of no avail in this disorder.

B. Alpha adrenergic blockers [Correct] lower blood pressure, and tachycardia is a problem with epinephrine-secreting tumors. Long acting Phenoxybenzamine hydrochloride or Doxazosin mesylate is used.

C. Beta blockers [Incorrect] are contraindicated as monotherapy, since the effect of alpha receptors would be unchallenged and hypertension would be exacerbated.

D. Angiotensin converting enzyme (ACE) inhibitors [Incorrect] are indicated in many hypertensive paradigms but not in hypertension associated with pheochromocytoma.

E. Though selective serotonin reuptake inhibitors [Incorrect] have an effect on vascular resistance, they are not an immediate treatment.

15-D

A. Fanconi anemia [Incorrect] is associated with macrocytosis and pancytopenia but not neutrophil hypersegmentation.

B. Vitamin B12 deficiency [Incorrect] purely due to diet is rare and can cause the megaloblastic anemia exhibited in this case.

Pernicious anemia with peripheral neuropathy is most often associated with a deficit in B12 or intrinsic factor and is not indicated in this case.

C. Vitamin E deficiency [Incorrect] may be seen in malabsorption syndromes but yields a low-grade hemolytic anemia.

D. The key is goats' milk, known to be deficient in folate [Correct], yielding the relatively rare megaloblastic anemia where cytoplasmic and RNA constituents are synthesized faster than their DNA counterparts since there is neither supplementation with breast milk, fortified milk, or cereals and baby food, all of which have adequate folate.

E. Iron deficiency [Incorrect] yields hypochromic, microcytic anemia.

16-B

Hint for genetics questions: draw a pedigree to determine the mode of inheritance!

A. Mitochondrial inheritance [Incorrect] is transmitted through mothers only, so no male-to-male inheritance.

B. Inheritance via autosomal dominant [Correct] exhibit the following: transmission from father-to-son, variable trait expression, a recurrence rate risk of 50%, reduced penetrance, and a significant spontaneous mutation rate.

C. Assuming no consanguinity, autosomal recessive [Incorrect] is very unlikely since there is transmission of the disorder through 3 generations of the family.

D. X-linked dominant [Incorrect] is excluded on the basis of male-to-male inheritance.

E. X-linked recessive [Incorrect] is excluded because females as well as males are affected in this family.

17-B

A. Hyperkalemia [Incorrect] would typically involve increased potassium intake, increased release of endogenous potassium, and decreased renal excretion in disorders such as rhabdomyolysis or multiple-degree burns.

B. With increased turnover of bone hypercalcemia [Correct] during repair and immobilization, this is the best possible answer. Over 98% of calcium in the body is in bone. The pool of free calcium, though small, is very tightly controlled, and homeostasis focuses on ionized calcium. Regulation proceeds through renal excretion/intestinal absorption by parathyroid hormone, vitamin D3, and calcitonin. Though hyperparathyroidism is the most common reason for hypercalcemia other reasons include: malignancy, idiopathic, or excess intake of calcium.

C. Hypocalcemia, [Incorrect] which stimulates PTH, is unexpected since there is increased turnover of bone upon repair and immobilization of bone.

D. Hypermagnesemia [Incorrect] would typically involve increased magnesium intake or decreased renal excretion of magnesium.

E. Hypomagnesemia [Incorrect] is associated with diarrhea with increased loss of magnesium, or renal excretion of magnesium such as in renal tubular acidosis.

18-B

General comment: a young infant presenting in the hospital with feeding difficulties, lethargy, and vomiting has a good probability of having an inborn error of metabolism. Physiologic hyperbilirubinemia is resolved within the first two weeks of life.

A. Cystic fibrosis [Incorrect] can be associated with elevated levels of conjugated bilirubin but the disease rarely presents itself in the neonatal period.

B. Consistent with classic galactosemia, [Correct] a lack of the enzyme Galactose-1-phosphate uridyl transferase catalyzing: galactose-1-P +UDP glucose → UDP galactose+glucose-1-P. An accumulation of toxic metabolites of galactose occurs with ingestion of human or cow milk, and synthetic formulas are used omitting this sugar.

C. As a disorder in amino acid metabolism, homocystinuria [Incorrect] is not associated with jaundice in infancy but with hepatic insufficiency in adolescence and Marfan-like changes.

D. Fructose intolerance [Incorrect] presents itself after the introduction of fructose, usually found in fruits and fruit juices.

E. Maple syrup urine disease [Incorrect] usually presents in the first week after birth with difficulty in feeding and then progresses rapidly to convulsions and muscle rigidity. Furthermore, there is no elevation of conjugated bilirubin or the smell of maple syrup in the urine.

19-E

Glycogen storage disease–Type I, also known as von Gierke disease, is a deficiency of glucose-6-phosphatatse inhibiting the conversion of glucose-6-phosphate to glucose. Hypoglycemia, hepatomegaly, and hyperuricemia are the first symptoms and usually present at nighttime with fasting and increased sleep.

The goal of long-term management is to avoid hypoglycemia and provide enough slowly released glucose.

A. Supplying medium chain triglycerides [Incorrect] is inconsequential and may lead to obesity.

B. L-carnitine [Incorrect] is administered in patients with fatty oxidation disorders and is of no aid in glycogen storage diseases.

C. There is no deficit in protein metabolism [Incorrect], so this will not alleviate the symptomology.

D. Chronic dextrose infusion [Incorrect] by an intravenous route is difficult to maintain.

E. Uncooked cornstarch [Correct] is the treatment of choice and provides a slow release of glucose from a complex carbohydrate.

20-E

A. Hunter syndrome [Incorrect] is an X-linked deficiency of iduronosulfate sulfatase deficiency that presents at 2 to 4 years of age with coarsening of facial features and developmental delay.

B. Hurler syndrome [Incorrect] presents after age 1 usually with a hernia, coarsening of facial features, short stature, cardiomegaly, corneal clouding, and developmental delays. This is a deficiency of alpha-iduronidase.

C. Niemann-Pick disease. [Incorrect] Sphingomyelin accumulates in Niemann-Pick disease, due to lack of sphingomyelinase. These patients exhibit hepatosplenomegaly and mental retardation. Progressive loss of vision and hearing may be seen.

D. Metachromatic leukodystrophy. [Incorrect] This disease is caused by deficiency of arylsulfatase A, leading to myelin breakdown. Accumulation of sulfatides causes demyelination, rather than galactocerebroside accumulation. Mental retardation is common. Affected patients die in the first decade of life.

E. Tay-Sachs disease. [Correct] Beta-hexosaminidase A deficiency is associated with mental retardation, blindness, seizures, and eventual paralysis. Ganglioside GM2 accumulates in the brain and presents at 4–6 months of age. Often, a cherry-red macula may be appreciated.

credits

Anderson SC. Anderson's Atlas of Hematology. Wolters Kluwer Health/Lippincott Williams & Wilkins, 2003. (Case 75).

Asset provided by Anatomical Chart Co. (Case 79).

Becker KL, Bilezikian JP, Brenner WJ, et al. Prinicples and Practice of Endocrinology and Metabolism, 3rd ed. Philadelphia: Lippincott Williams & Wilkins, 2001. Figs. 163-4 (Case 2), 70-2 (Case 6), 115-12 (Case 13), 90-23A (Case 17), 153-7 (Case 21), 88-7 (Case 22), 80-10 (Case 26), 68-3 (Case 27), 158-3 (Case 30), 159-2 (Case 31), 115-16A&B (Case 32), 60-2 (Case 36), 88-5A (Case 37), 192-5 (Case 65).

Bhushan V, Le T, Pall V. Underground Clinical Vignettes: Step 1 Biochemistry, 4th ed. Malden, Massachusetts: Blackwell Publishing, 2005. Figs. 89 (Case 70), 93 (Case 85), 95 (Case 100).

Bucholz RW, Heckman JD. Rockwood & Green's Fractures in Adults, 5th ed. Philadelphia: Lippincott Williams & Wilkins, 2001. Fig. 41.33C (Case 35).

Champe PC, Harvery RA, Ferrier DR. Lippincott's Illustrated Reviews: Biochemistry, 3rd ed. Philadelphia: Lippincott Wilkins & Williams, 2004. Figs. 28.19 (Cases 7 & 8), 28.27 (Case 12), 22.21 (Case 69), 20.15 (Case 71), 29.28 (Case 78), 23.15 (Case 91), 3.12 (Case 96), 3.8 (Case 98).

Crocett M, Barone MA. Oski's Essential Pediatrics, 2nd ed. Philadelphia: Lippincott Williams & Wilkins, 2004. Figs. Table 205-1 (Case 38), p. 730 (Case 53), p. 724 (Cases 56 & 63), 216-4 (Case 61), 224-1 (Case 64).

Eisenberg RL. Clinical Imaging: An Atlas of Differential Diagnosis. 4th ed. Philadelphia: Lippincott Williams & Wilkins. Fig. GU 15-1A (Case 52).

Fleisher GR, Ludwig S, Baskin MN. Atlas of Pediatric Emergency Medicine. Phildelphia: Lippincott Williams & Wilkins, 2004. Fig. 16.2 (Case 95)

Goodheart HP. Goodheart's Photoguide of Common Skin Disorders, 2nd ed. Philadelphia: Lippincott Williams & Wilkins, 2003. Fig. 11.2 (Case 29).

Greenberg MJ, Hendrickson RG. Greenberg's Text-Atlas of Emergency Medicine. Philadelphia: Lippincott, Williams & Wilkins, 2004. Figs. 22-6A (Case 25), 24-13B (Case 88).

Greer JP, Foerster J, Lukens J, et al. Wintrobe's Clinical Hematology, 11th ed. Philadelphia: Lippincott Williams & Wilkins, 1998. Figs. 65.3 (Case 58), 65.4 (Case 68), 27.21 (Case 87).

Humes HD, DuPont HL, Gardner LB, et al. Kelley's Textbook of Internal Medicine, 4th ed. Philadelphia: Lippincott Williams & Wilkins, 2000. Tables 103.1 (Cases 45 & 47), 155.1 (Case 89).

Stedman's Medical Dictionary, 27th ed. Baltimore: Lippincott Williams & Wilkins, 2003. (Case 74).

Koopman WJ, Moreland LW. Arthritis and Allied Conditions: A Textbook of Rheumatology, 15th ed. Philadelphia: Lippincott Williams & Wilkins, 2004. Fig. 120.5 (Case 50).

Lee G, Foerster J, Lukens J, et al. Wintrobe's Clinical Hematology, 10th ed. Philadelphia: Lippincott Williams & Wilkins, 1998. Figs. 10.17 (Case 85), 10.2D (Case 83), 10.4B (Case 82).

McClatchey KD. Clinical Laboratory Medicine, 2nd ed. Philadelphia: Lippincott Williams & Wilkins, 2002. Fig. 41.10 (Case 81)

McMillan JA, Fergin RD, et al. Oski's Pediatrics: Principles and Practice. 4th ed. Philadelphia: Lippincott Williams & Wilkins, 2006. Figs. 128.26 (Case 49), 389.15 (Case 54), 385.4A (Case 60), 289.6A (Case 62), 387.2 (Case 77), 270.2 (Case 99).

Menkes JH, Sarnat HB, Maria BL. Child Neurology, 7th ed. Philadelphia: Lippincott Williams & Wilkins, 2005. Fig. 1.30 (Case 48).

Nyberg DA, McGahan JD, Pretorius DH, Pilu G. Diagnostic Imaging of Fetal Anomalies. Philadelphia: Lippincott, Williams & Wilkins, 2002. Fig. 53B (Case 55).

Porth CM. Pathophysiology Concepts in Altered Health States, 6th ed. Philadelphia: Lippincott Williams & Wilkins, 2002. From Chapter 6 (Case 15).

Rowland LP. Merritt's Neurology, 11th ed. Philadelphia: Lippincott Williams & Wilkins, 2005. Figs. 84.4 (Case 76), 154.2 (Case 87).

Rubin E, Farber JL. Pathology, 3rd ed. Philadelphia: Lippincott Williams & Wilkins, 1999. Figs. 8.29 (Case 7), 6.21 (Case 51).

Rubin E, Gorstein F, Schwarting R, et al. Rubin's Pathology: A Clinicopathologic Approach. 4th ed. Baltimore: Lippincott Williams & Wilkins, 2004. Figs. 8-33 (Case 11), 21-28 (Case 24), 21-25 (Case 39), 14-6 (Case 46), 16-69 (Case 92), 28-115A (Case 94).

Schiff ER, Sorrell MF, Maddrey WC. Schiff's Diseases of the Liver, 9th ed. Philadelphia: Lippincott Williams & Wilkins. Table 44.2 (Case 43).

Smith C, Marks A, Lieberman M. Mark's Basic Medical Biochemistry: A Clinical Approach, 2nd ed. Philadelphia: Lippincott Williams & Wilkins, 2004. Figs. 22.15 (Case 3), 34.23 (Case 14), 39.15 (Case 66), 31.7A (Case 72).

case list

CARDIOLOGY/CARDIOVASCULAR

1. Familial Hypercholesterolemia
2. Familial Hypertriglyceridemia
3. Lactic Acidosis
4. Pesticide (Organophosphate) Poisoning

NUTRITION

5. Kwashiorkor
6. Rickets
7. Vitamin A Deficiency
8. Vitamin A Toxicity
9. Vitamin B_1 Deficiency (Beriberi)
10. Pellagra
11. Vitamin C Deficiency (Scurvy)
12. Vitamin K Deficiency

ENDOCRINOLOGY

13. 5-α-Reductase Deficiency
14. 17-α-Hydroxylase Deficiency
15. Acromegaly
16. Addison Disease
17. Androgen Insensitivity Syndrome
18. Bartter Syndrome
19. Diabetic Ketoacidosis
20. Diabetes Insipidus
21. Glucagonoma
22. Hyperaldosteronism—Primary
23. Hypercalcemia
24. Hyperparathyroidism—Primary
25. Hyperthyroidism (Graves Disease)
26. Hypokalemia
27. Hypomagnesemia
28. Hyponatremia
29. Hirsutism—Idiopathic
30. Insulin Overdose
31. Insulinoma
32. Kallmann Syndrome
33. Metabolic Alkalosis
34. Nonketotic Hyperosmolar Coma
35. Osteomalacia
36. Pancreatic Hypocalcemia
37. Pheochromocytoma
38. Precocious Puberty
39. Pseudohypoparathyroidism
40. SIADH—Syndrome of Inappropriate Antidiuretic Hormone Secretion
41. Testosterone Deficiency
42. Thyroid Storm

GASTROENTEROLOGY

43. Acute Intermittent Porphyria
44. Carcinoid Syndrome
45. Crigler–Najjar Syndrome
46. Dubin–Johnson Syndrome
47. Gilbert Disease
48. Wilson Disease

GENETICS

49. Albinism
50. Alkaptonuria
51. Cystic Fibrosis
52. Cystinuria
53. Ehlers–Danlos Syndrome
54. Fabry Disease
55. Fanconi Anemia
56. Fragile X Syndrome
57. Galactosemia
58. Gaucher Disease
59. Hereditary Fructose Intolerance
60. Homocystinuria

61. Hunter Disease
62. Hurler Disease
63. Klinefelter Syndrome
64. Krabbe Disease
65. Lesch–Nyhan Syndrome
66. Maple Syrup Urine Disease
67. Metachromatic Leukodystrophy
68. Niemann–Pick Disease
69. Orotic Aciduria
70. Osteogenesis Imperfecta
71. Phenylketonuria (PKU)
72. Phosphoenolpyruvate Carboxykinase Deficiency
73. Pompe Disease
74. Porphyria Cutanea Tarda
75. Pyruvate Kinase Deficiency
76. Tay–Sachs Disease
77. von Gierke Disease
78. Xeroderma Pigmentosum

GYNECOLOGY

79. Secondary Amenorrhea

HEMATOLOGY

80. Folate Deficiency Anemia
81. Glucose-6-Phosphate Dehydrogenase Deficiency
82. Hemophilia
83. Hereditary Spherocytosis
84. Iron Deficiency Anemia
85. Methemoglobinemia
86. Paroxysmal Nocturnal Hemoglobinuria
87. Vitamin B_{12} Deficiency

NEPHROLOGY/UROLOGY

88. Ethylene Glycol Ingestion
89. Renal Tubular Acidosis
90. Rhabdomyolysis

NEUROLOGY/PSYCHIATRY

91. Antabuse Effect (Disulfiram-like Reaction)
92. Mercury Toxicity
93. Duchenne Muscular Dystrophy
94. Wernicke–Korsakoff Syndrome

PULMONARY

95. Alpha-1-Antitrypsin Deficiency
96. Carbon Monoxide Poisoning
97. Hyaline Membrane Disease
98. Hyperventilation
99. Kartagener Syndrome

RHEUMATOLOGY

100. Gout

index